THE CENTER OF TANTRIC SEX

A DISTINCTIVE GUIDE TO LOVE AND SEXUAL SUCCESS

John K. Hall

TABLE OF CONTENTS

INTRODUCTION

I REMEMBER BEING OVERWHELMED WITH DISAPPOINTMENT THE FIRST TIME I MADE LOVE, especially because I had waited for love and made it a special event. I questioned, "Is this the cause of all the commotion? There must be more to it, right?"

Even though I was able to establish what some might consider a healthy sex life after my first encounter, I have always felt that there must be more to sex—especially given the stigma attached to it and the numerous laws and norms that surround sexual conduct. I've always liked having sex, but I've never been very touched. I wasn't as engrossed or interested as I had anticipated being.

I decided to start a genuine investigation into the enigmatic subject of sex when I realized that, after having made love several times, I still didn't grasp how sexual energy worked. It was the sporadic moments of love in my life that stood out as clearly distinct from the others as to what drove me in my research and kept me going when I felt disheartened. As they happened, time seemed to halt, and space and the air around me seemed to expand to expose a new level of sensory awareness. It appeared as though an inner bodily intellect seized over and I became instantly genuinely alive. I had no idea how or why this occurred, but it gave me hope that there was a fundamental truth about sex that I still needed to learn.

I now understand I'm not alone. I have seen many people who are experiencing the same frustrations and asking themselves the same questions via my considerable work with couples over the years. They are caught in a loop that is repeated every time they make love, and it seldom ever involves anything original or novel, just like I was. Eventually, boredom and disinterest set in.

Although many others frequently switch partners to make sex hot and intriguing, some will experiment with provocative costumes and movies. Even yet, this rarely provides long-lasting satisfaction. While a couple may still be in love, the sexual desire frequently fades and they cease physically expressing their affection for one another. They could even find themselves opting to split up at some point. But despite this, we continue to look for this manifestation of love because we have a strong need that never really goes away.

After conducting extensive research for many years, I found that the Tantric experience—which involves relaxing into sex energy rather than exerting pressure on it—was what provided me the intuitive fulfillment I had yearned for my whole life. It was like discovering a set of keys that opened one door after another. My spirit was affected by the process of learning long-kept truths regarding sexual energy, which led to an unanticipated sense of inner calm.

To have a fulfilling experience of sex and love, one had to gradually learn an entirely new language. With the use of this language, I was introduced to a brand-new, distinctive universe where the sexual rut vanished and inventiveness grew. I discovered that many of my beliefs about sex were impeding my progress and that I had to unlearn the old language to master the new. It took me many months to sort through the misconceptions society had given me and to discover a calm place free from the strain of the orgasm, which I had mistakenly thought was the point of sex.

Once upon a time, in a quaint little village nestled amidst rolling hills, lived a couple named Maya and Ravi. They had been married for several years and had always shared a deep love and respect for one another. However, as time went by, the responsibilities and stresses of daily life began to take a toll on their intimate connection.

Feeling a sense of longing for the passion and fire they once had, Maya decided to embark on a journey of self-discovery. She had heard whispers about the ancient practice of tantric sex—a path that promised to unlock hidden realms of pleasure and connection between couples.

Filled with curiosity and a desire to reignite the spark in their marriage, Maya approached Ravi one evening with a proposition. She explained her findings and suggested that they explore tantric practices together. Intrigued by the idea, Ravi agreed, and thus began their transformative journey.

The couple sought out a wise and experienced tantric teacher who resided on the outskirts of the village. The teacher, named Guruji, welcomed them warmly and sensed the sincerity of their intention. He understood that their relationship was in need of a spiritual revival, and he decided to guide them on their path.

Under Guruji's tutelage, Maya and Ravi began to learn the intricacies of tantric sex. They discovered that it was more than just a physical act; it was a practice that involved deepening their emotional connection, harnessing their energy, and opening their hearts to one another.

In their first session, Guruji taught them about the power of breath. They learned to synchronize their breathing, allowing it to flow in unison and create a harmonious rhythm between them. As they breathed together, a profound sense of intimacy and unity blossomed within their beings.

In subsequent sessions, Guruji introduced them to the art of touch. They explored the concept of mindful caresses, where every stroke was performed with intention and presence. Through this practice, they rediscovered the pleasure of simply being in each other's arms and feeling the warmth and tenderness of their touch.

As Maya and Ravi delved deeper into tantric practices, they uncovered the importance of communication. They discovered the beauty of expressing their desires and fantasies, without judgment or inhibition. Through honest and open conversations, they created a safe space for vulnerability, where their deepest desires and fears could be shared without reservation.

With each passing day, Maya and Ravi noticed a remarkable transformation in their marriage. The once-dormant embers of passion were reignited into a blazing fire of desire. They found themselves longing for one another, eagerly exploring new realms of pleasure, and connecting on levels they had never experienced before.

Tantric sex had become a sacred ritual for them, a way to honor their love and celebrate their union. It was no longer just about physical satisfaction but a profound union of mind, body, and soul. Their journey had awakened a new dimension in their relationship, creating a blissful and fulfilling marriage.

Maya and Ravi's newfound connection spilled over into every aspect of their lives. They approached their daily tasks with renewed enthusiasm, and their bond as a couple grew stronger than ever. They became a beacon of love and inspiration for those around them, as others witnessed the radiant glow that emanated from their transformed marriage.

Their story spread far and wide, inspiring many other couples to embark on their own tantric journeys. The power of tantric sex became a catalyst for rekindling passion, deepening connections, and enjoying the profound beauty of marriage.

And so, Maya and Ravi continued to live their days with a twinkle in their eyes and hearts full of love, forever grateful for the gift of tantric sex that had transformed their lives and allowed them to experience the true magic of marriage.

The main problem for couples nowadays is how to keep their relationship new and exciting. How can we strengthen and expand this love, after all? Tantra provides solutions that have the impact of boosting closeness and fostering a deeper level of love via its singular and perceptive approach to sex. Tantra, which encourages relaxation and relieves many sex-related stresses, surprisingly provides us with greater joy and contentment. In our deepest selves, so many of us want this, but we just don't know how to make it happen.

My friend was facing a difficult situation. He was deeply conflicted over which of the two ladies he was in love with to select, and he was in pain and suffering. He saw a therapist, who questioned him about who he preferred to make love to more.

Cathy, he uttered.

She said, "Then go with Cathy."

I was in a long-term relationship where sex had lost its excitement and passion when my buddy first told me this tale, so I was unable to comprehend the therapist's response. I now do. I've discovered that the likelihood of a loving relationship and happy marriage increases anytime sex is satisfying. Sexual chemistry opens the door to sincerity, closeness, and a solidifying, loving partnership. In contrast, when there is unhappiness in the bedroom, the seeds of unhappiness are sowed, resentments, disappointments, and worries quickly emerge, and gradually the love and chemistry between couples can deteriorate, eventually leading to separation.

Because of the extreme ignorance in our society, it appears normal for young people to be battling in ignorance while attempting to capture sexual energy, the essential power of life. Early in childhood, we often pay a high price for poor sexual encounters or ill-informed assumptions; these memories stick with us and impact us every day. Insecurity and a lack of trust may turn intimate relations into a nightmare. Tantra is an antidote, reeducation in sex, and education that our parents, grandparents, and great-grandparents never received. Tantra is an old art.

Tantra experimentation has gradually taught me a new way of making love that has transformed not just my sex life but also my experience of love, and hence life itself, much more meaningful. I used to feel as if I was swimming in shallow water, unaware of what my purpose in life was, what to do, and how to be.

My life took on a new perspective, and I felt as though I was returning home as my boyfriend and I embraced the Tantric teachings, piercing the deeper seas of sex and the heightened love that emerged from it. I now realize that sex serves as a means for me to connect with my innermost self, my inner world, and my quiet self since the roots of genuine satisfaction do not reside outside of me. I now have a lot more depth and substance than I ever could have with my goals and accomplishments alone.

Tantra teaches us that sex is the foundation of real relaxation. Regrettably, in most facets of our culture, we have lost the skill of relaxing. And for many of us, sex, in particular, has turned into a cause of worry and anxiety. Many of the concerns and tensions that we have been conditioned to have about sex will automatically dissipate as we start to relax during the sexual act. If we can unwind into the sex energy, the inner calm it creates will radiate out, bringing the same sense of peace and loving ease to the rest of life.

When we experiment with sex, we get more intimate with both our partners and our bodies and sexualities. With this comes an acceptance of the simple truth, with nothing hidden, that nakedness is sacred. And out of this arises confidence based on self-understanding. Through the experience of Tantra, we find that what we have always hoped is true: love and joy can be a tangible reality for each of us, not an impossible dream.

Two primary sources made this dream possible for me. My years of experience and inspiration are based on two audio tapes entitled "Making Love" produced by Barry Long. In these discourses, he offers revolutionary insight into men and women and a completely different perspective on love and lovemaking. At first, in my ignorance, I was too proud to admit that I did not know, in truth, how to make love. I returned to these teachings some five years later, during which time I felt I had exhausted the routine of sex. But now my attitude has changed.

I listened to the tapes in gratitude, knowing there was something I did not yet know about love and sex. The depth and detail of the information given by Barry Long changed the course of my life. Through ongoing experimentation within the specific guidelines, I was able to face and challenge my sexual conditioning. This essential groundwork gave me the experience of discovering a new "genital connection." Furthermore, it enabled me to understand and absorb, in a bodily way, the words of my spiritual master, Osho. He includes a vision of spirituality through sex, woven together with interpretations of the ancient Tantric scriptures, which were born in India thousands of years ago.

These words remain a treasure for humanity today. Both of these sources represent Tantric teaching at its highest level.

This book is an attempt to share practical information about sex that has created a subtle and significant revolution in my life. It is by no means intended to be a comprehensive presentation of the origins or intricate esoteric aspects of Tantra; it is simply a personal experience. The material appears in three sections: "The Roots" looks at the divine potential of sex and love; "The Love Keys" offers practical body-oriented suggestions; and "The Journey" delves into crucial aspects of sex and sexuality. Sex is a vast subject, and even while attempting to streamline the information, the different themes naturally link and interweave.

Reading "The Love Keys" again and again, in conjunction with your own experiences while using them, will bring you deeper insights into sex, support your exploration, and strengthen your perception.

CHAPTER ONE

THE ROOTS

INSPIRATION

THE MALE BODY AND THE FEMALE BODY ARE SIMILAR, but still, different in many, many ways. And the difference is always complimentary. Whatever is positive in the male body will be negative in the female body, and whatever is positive in the female body will be negative in the male body. That is why when they meet in deep orgasms, they become one organism. The positive meets the negative, the negative meets the positive, and both become—one circle of electricity. Hence so much attraction for sex, so much appeal. This appeal is not because man is a sinner or immoral, it is not because the modern world has become too licentious; it is not because of obscene films and literature—it is very deep-rooted, very cosmic.

The attraction is because both males and females are half circuits, and there is an inherent tendency in existence to transcend whatever is incomplete and to become complete. This is one of the ultimate laws —the tendency towards completion. Nature abhors incompleteness, any type of incompleteness. The male is incomplete, the female is incomplete, and they can have only one moment of completion—when their electrical circuits become one when the two are dissolved. That is why the two most important words in all languages are love and prayer. In love, you become one with a single individual; in prayer, you become one with the whole cosmos. And love and prayer are similar as far as their inner workings are concerned.

REFRAMING SEX

SEX ATTRACTS EVERYONE'S ATTENTION. That is the one topic that has persisted through the ages as a source of unending intrigue if not obsession. When sex is the topic of a conversation, you can tell right once because heads move nearby and the atmosphere becomes somber and intense. But there can be a distinct sense of separation, a barrier of isolation and tension around people who are ashamed of or afraid to talk about sex or of sex and its "animal" nature. The fact is that sex is the most important component of our life, regardless of whether it is discussed or avoided, expressed or suppressed, or loved or suffered.

Sex is constantly on the brain. It is a major theme in our daydreams and thoughts. Since every sentient being on this planet was produced in sex through the union of male and female cells, it is a natural element of our chemistry. When we naturally fondle our genitalia with innocent comforting delight as children, we first become aware of this. Our sexuality then follows us throughout our lives in various stages of development and expression. It is the cause of a lot of pleasure and discomfort as well as anguish. It frequently dictates our joys and sorrows, ecstasies and agonies.

We can start attracting sex by doing something as easy as painting our toes or lips or applying perfume or aftershave. Today, when we are continuously exposed to sexually explicit words, images, and videos, this is very clear. People use sex to control, entice, abuse, and abandon, while the media uses it to market, humiliate, and scandalize. Our preoccupation with looks and fashion has a lot to do with sex.

Even if we don't think they're very gorgeous, it makes us feel alive and confident to be thought of as attractive. We feel excited when we glimpse the possibility of love when desires are shared. To love and be loved is what each of us longs for. Nothing can ever replace it. And when we love someone, having sex with them continues to be a kind of communication.

Moreover, sex can be the root of misunderstandings, fights, aggression, uncertainty, unhappiness, and restlessness. Men are rumored to think about sex every three minutes, while women do so every six to seven. Whether we like it or not, the reality that we as human beings are in a continual connection with sex, regardless of the actual figures, cannot be denied.

Sexual Energy And The Life Force

Sexual energy cannot be contained since it is the very essence of existence. Although we frequently attempt to distinguish between sexual energy and "other" energy in our brains, the reality is that they are all the same. Energy is just energy with the ability to move, and it moves regardless of how the life force manifests itself—through sex or survival, in art, sport, or music. And despite our best efforts, we are powerless to suppress or dismiss this energy; all we can do is learn to use it in the wisest and most uplifting manner possible.

Despite how common sex is, very few people have figured out how to obtain complete satisfaction or a loving heart from engaging in it. An "average" sexually active person feels orgasmic bliss for twenty seconds each week, ninety seconds per month, or eighteen minutes per year, according to current studies on the topic. And this is predicated on a ten-second orgasm. Ten seconds alone can seem like quite an accomplishment! We thus have the luxury of enjoying orgasmic ecstasy for a total of fifteen hours during fifty years of sexual engagement. When you consider how frequently you have intimate encounters and how much more time is spent daydreaming and experiencing agony over them, this is startling (and distressing).

For the majority of us, love and sex are not satisfactory. Sex is not the spiritual, pure, orgasmic power that it is supposed to be, bringing us into a world of love and genuine desire. It neither deeply satisfies us, giving us the willpower to face each day with enthusiasm, nor does it have the capacity to lift us above the constraints or pressures of our daily lives. Sexual abuse, frigidity, ambivalence, premature ejaculation, impotence, and sexual apathy are all frequent sexual issues that affect men and women.

Sex And Intelligence

We need to start integrating intellect into our conception of sex to turn this around and get the depth of sexual enjoyment we seek. To approach it from a fresh angle and inside a new framework what we must do? Beyond reproduction or short-term bodily enjoyment, we must look. With this new perspective, we will get a new understanding of sexual energy, how it responds, and how to make the most of sex as a living expression of love between men and women. And the good news is that we may benefit much from and enjoy sex, which is a very healthy and empowering force.

In its purest form, sex contains a divine aspect. It transports you to "here," where you are blissfully at ease in the divinity of the present moment.

The pieces are all precisely in place. It is food for the spirit because it is an ecstatic biological delight that results from the dynamic interaction of opposing forces. Regrettably, a lot of religious people believe that sexual activity is a deterrent on the road to God. Some of us have been trained to "avoid sex at all costs," even if we dream erratically at night and incessantly think about it throughout the day.

This is a grave mistake that causes humanity to suffer greatly. Our life energy is lost if sex is restricted to reproduction and immediate enjoyment and its delicate spiritual purpose is disregarded, upsetting the mind, body, and spirit. Through Tantra, the cosmic balancing of yin and yang, positive and negative, dynamic and receptive, masculine and female energies, we can incorporate love and spirit in our lives, both internally and externally, and learn to transcend the bounds of straightforward biology. By the physical act of making love, we are given the chance to rediscover our true selves as men and women and to learn the spiritual language of love. It depicts sex differently than the one we were raised with. Tantra offers us fresh perspectives and an entirely other understanding of sex and its purpose.

Phases Of Sexual Energy

It is believed that sexual energy in humans travels in a circular pattern along internal pathways with two separate phases.

The brain serves as the first stage and initial drive of sexual energy before it circles down to the genitals (see fig. 1). More specifically, the brain's pineal gland and hypothalamic-pituitary area secrete hormones that regulate the endocrine system, which includes the sex glands.

These hormones support ongoing sexual health and eventual preparation for sexual activity. From the brain to the genitalia, this is the first and descending part of the circle. The biological or reproductive phase of sexual energy is referred to as this.

And it is at this point that we almost always ejaculate or have an orgasm to release the sexual energy
that is created during sex.

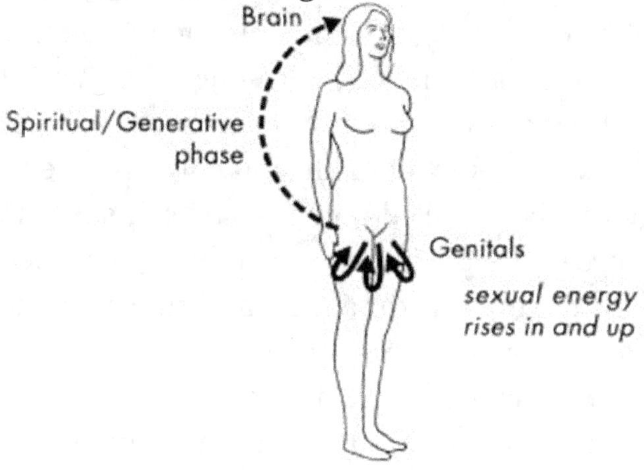

Fig. 2   Spiritual or generative phase of sexual energy

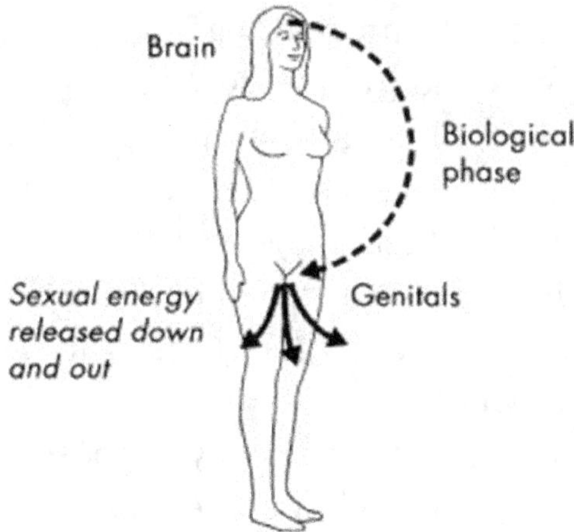

Fig. 1   Biological or reproductive phase of sexual energy

Sexual energy is urged to be preserved in the body, which is the secret of Tantra and its main focus. It does not frequently come out during orgasm or ejaculation. We reach our orgasmic potential by having it stay inside the body and be recirculated. Sexual energy has the chance to return to the brain, where it originated, during this second half and rising phase, revitalizing and nourishing the body's "master" glands (pituitary and pineal).

The health of these glands is significantly impacted. Sexual activity is known to release a variety of hormones that have a good impact on both the body and the mind, and from ancient times, sex has been linked to elongated life and enlightenment. When sexual energy can be recycled and reabsorbed, sex acts as a reinvigorating force. The genitals are reverently regarded as reproductive organs during this time, which is known as the spiritual or generative phase of sex (see fig. 2).

Tantra's insight is that we can access this second stage of our sexual energy by letting it spiral upward and inward. It demonstrates to us that sex may be used to produce more life rather than just another life.

As men and women learn to unwind together during sex, this spiritual phase of sexual energy emerges. Contrary to popular belief, sex is not an effort but rather a pressure-filled action. We think that the more sexual activity we engage in, the more things will occur and the higher the payoff. We barely ever consider relaxing! We fail to recognize the connection between genuine sexual enjoyment and bodily relaxation. We feel better the more we unwind.

Ecstasy and tension are diametrically opposed; whereas tension results in heat and agitation, ecstasy springs from coolness and inner tranquility. While relaxation opens and expands, tension closes and narrows. Tension forces a release, whereas relaxation permits absorption. Tension creates a peak, while relaxation creates a valley.

The entire atmosphere of Tantra is one of relaxation. It implies that more life energy and more love will result when we relax into our sexual energy rather than raising it to a peak and then releasing it. We can convert sexual energy inward and upward by relaxing, which will cause it to be immediately reabsorbed by the body and circulated (see fig. 3). This action is described in the Tantra as putting a foot on the bottom rung of the inner staircase of progress. It takes some time for a body's core to develop a neglected energy conduit, but once it does, we feel wonderful golden light phenomena rising from the genitalia up. Lovemaking turns into a divine experience full of wonder when we support the spiritual phase of sex rather than hindering it as we do in

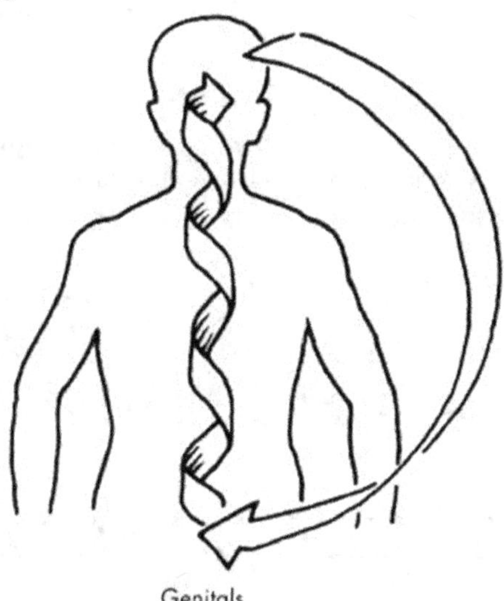

Fig. 3   Complete sexual energy circle, with redirected sexual energy spiraling through energy centers

ignorance.

❚❚ Sexual energy is the life force itself running through us all.

❚❚ By balancing our male and female energies we can enjoy a healthy, empowering sexual relationship.

❚❚ We can direct sexual energy in the usual way by orgasm or we can redirect it to give us more energy, more love.

❚❚ Sex is transformed creatively into a truly uplifting experience.

Notes

1. The Art of Sexual Ecstasy, Margo Anand, page 347 (quoting from ESO by Alan P Brauer & Donna J. Brauer).
2. Sexual Energy Ecstasy by David & Ellen Ramsdale, pages 118—121.

CHAPTER TWO

SEXUAL CONDITIONING

If sex is such a fundamental aspect of human nature, how did we lose sight of its more pleasurable potential? How did we forget how to make people fall in love? of remaining devoted? Why do we care so much about orgasm? Sadly, the straightforward explanation is that as we have advanced in civilization, we have lost consciousness. Over thousands of years, men and women have become significantly out of balance with one another. We've gotten more and more time- and goal-focused, which makes it harder to have genuine love and uplifting sex.

With the advancement of technology, we have developed an addiction to time, accomplishments, plans, and achieving our objectives, no matter what they may be. Time becomes more crucial when a nation develops because more people live busy lives with back-to-back appointments. This puts so much strain on us that we not only lose our capacity for love but also end up being sick. In the current world, stress is thought to be the cause of a very high percentage of illnesses.

We are so unaccustomed to calmness and inner ease that we get restless and bored when we aren't "doing" anything. Humans want movement, thrills, and stimulation. It appears that we have turned the natural order on its head. While "being" and silence and calm make us anxious, living with and against the clock seems to give our life significance.

Why Are We So Goal-Oriented In Sex?

How frequently have you said to yourself or your partner, "I want to get intimate? I simply lack the time." That is accurate in a sense since fulfilling sex takes time. But, when we do make love, we always want to get to the orgasmic portion right away. We are moving ahead of ourselves when we are working toward that. We are not truly "here," and we are not truly even present as a group. Our every action or contact is directed at achieving our aim, and we are almost using each other. We feel that sex is not truly sex until we "come," unless there is a peak and release of energy, and the orgasm has become the sole way to do this. In our experience, millions of women worry and suffer emotionally when they are unable to have the illusive orgasm, and the majority of men are disturbed because they ejaculate much earlier than they would like—or at the very least, much earlier than they can please their partner. We feel that we are lacking something, that we have failed, or that we are sexually insufficient unless we "come together."

Our unconscious desire for an orgasm practically acts as an involuntary reaction, giving us little choice except to proceed with our regular orgasmic behavior. It is even more difficult for us to believe there might be alternative methods to make love because this need is so intense it seems to be instinctual. To reach a particular contentment that we never seem to find, we repeat ourselves in sex.

Together with religious dogma, this goal-oriented tendency has been suppressing our sexual energy for centuries. It causes hasty sex and has been linked to centuries of goal orientation. Our enjoyment of orgasm and sex is restricted by a variety of concerns, uncertainties, anxieties, tensions, and pressures that we are exposed to, all of which are kept hidden from us.

We no longer know that there are other ways to make love, and the way that we express our sexual energy is now constrained by certain rules that force us to take a particular sexual path from beginning to end. It almost feels like a routine. Because my mother, grandmother, and great-grandmother made love in this manner, and if it was good enough for them, why not me? these conditions sadly exist without our knowledge. That's what I believed up until I started looking at love from a different perspective.

From Doing To Being

The result is that we are no longer able to learn how the genitals themselves "make love" or what they "want to do" since we are directing the sexual energy toward achieving a certain aim. We already know exactly what we want. Due to the unintentional loss of our "organic genital intelligence," sex nowadays is a mental activity rather than a bodily one. A biological and extroverted approach to sex has resulted from this sexual programming. Our bodies have gotten too tense and our sexual energy has become congested as a result. Our lifelong practice of constricting sexual energy and directing it—intentionally or unintentionally—along a predetermined, goal-oriented path has caused it to twist in an almost "nearly corkscrew" fashion. The genital organs are tense and considerably less sensitive than they should be because of the physical and mental tensions that have built up inside us as a result of our past experiences. We no longer have access to the heavenly "being" components of sexual union, and sex is more of a mechanical "doing" and reproductive purpose. We don't understand how to "be" in love; we only know how to "do" it.

Imagine a flower that is constricted, confined, and never given the chance to open and bloom. We are in this situation. Chronic tension prevents the body's naturally expansive energy from spreading throughout it because the sexual center is twisted and turned in on itself. We lose the ability to produce greater euphoric experiences, and sex is reduced to local genital feelings.

Once bodies and genitals relax and are no longer pushed by orgasm, the inward and upward swing of sex energy necessary by Tantra occurs, and that same energy spreads and expands delectably throughout the body. Nevertheless, very few of us have had this experience because when we try to manage and control the path of sex energy, we just get far too tense. When the same energy is allowed to move completely on its own, sex transforms into a wonderful fusion of raging passion and somber silence.

Personal psychology and programming

Individual psychologies and personalities are housed in the sexual center. We get our programming from places like these. Here, long before we engage in sexual activity, are stored our initial, unconscious thoughts about sex and life, which continue to influence us for the rest of our lives. While we are still young, bad impressions, and millennia of sexual misconceptions, phrases, and glances infiltrate our bodies. This is how our sexual programming is passed on to us; it manifests in the body as physical tension and a restless, agitated aspect. The tensions from our shared history compound the tensions from our past, which may be conscious or not.

Excitement and sexual tension

The unconscious tension within each of us is triggered to develop an urgent physical desire as soon as our degree of sexual arousal reaches a particular point, which sets up a powerful longing for the climax. We instantly depart from the present moment after this abrupt buildup of tension as we race madly toward an unnatural climax brought on by a concentration on the future. In actuality, we are not present during sex because we are seeking a particular result.

In this perspective, sexual energy is no longer a motivating and empowering force, but rather a delightful accumulation and release of stress. However, this sexual tension rarely totally leaves or exits the body. Instead, it persists as a disappointed desire that builds up over time and is constantly looking for an outlet. It causes us to feel emotional, restless, lustful, or angry while also making our genitals tough and insensitive. Sexual stimulation causes this built-up tension to be ignited or propelled ahead, which disturbs the already unstable energy in the sexual center.

Similar to a building's foundation, all the above structures will lack strength and support from the earth if the base is weak. The body's higher energy centers will likewise lack vitality, nutrition, and purity similarly. As a result, a system that is already frail at the core may collapse when the tensions of obtaining orgasm are the central focus of lovemaking.

The entire collective unconscious surrounding sex will automatically hook and mobilize when the vulnerable sex center is pulled or given a corkscrew twist. The purity and spirituality of sexual activity are lost when the torrent of psychological disorders and perversions that have developed through thousands of years seep through to us now. While it manifests in the body, this is essentially a mental illness; even though it manifests in the body.

Time for relaxation

Tantra realigns us with our fundamentally sexual nature to immediately treat the mind and the restlessness of the psyche. One facet of the spirit is sex. The recent resurgence of interest in traditional sexual attitudes and practices is an honest effort to stem the tide of sexual ignorance because today's sexual act has little to do with heart and soul. We start to break our ties with our conditioned personal and collective pasts and open up to a new realm of experience by bringing intellect into sex, by experiencing sexual energy in an innocent, playful, childlike way, absorbed beyond any concern about outcome.

Time is what we make of it, therefore to start, we need to have a flexible attitude about it. Time puts pressure on us to cram more into our days and accomplish more tasks if time equals money. When time flows in cycles, as it does in nature, patience is a virtue that relieves stress and replaces it with ease. Some plants need to wait years for rains so they may bloom for only a few short hours.

Have you ever wondered how in the world you would finish everything, only to find yourself suddenly on an aircraft, flying away, with everything planned out and in its proper place? If time is what we make it to be, it must be adaptable enough that it can even stop. Tantra begs for a patient, compassionate approach since this occurs as we enter the present moment. We become aware of the rich present moment that is unfolding when we are not rushing or worried about the passing of time. While I was in India, I noticed that time was essentially meaningless and that no one gave a damn about it.

The past, present, or future didn't matter. It's interesting to note that in Hindi, yesterday and tomorrow are both described by the same word, "kal"! A sense of being rather than doing was given to the entire nation by this perspective on time. A crowded train can stop and remain motionless for five hours at the end of a five-hour journey when it is only 20 minutes from its destination, as happened to mine.

The cause of the delay was not disclosed. When this occurred to me, the other passengers just sat silently; nothing was said or done, and everyone instantly and joyfully accepted what had transpired. Spicy delicacies started to come, adults relaxed and spoke, kids played and walked around the cramped compartment as if they were at home, and gradually the train started moving again.

There was no commotion or panic because nobody had a deadline for getting somewhere.

I remember flying on a German jet from Frankfurt to Berlin after returning to Europe after spending several years living in India. The young businessman next to me was agitated since the departure was already running late and kept looking at his watch. He was furious that life's difficulties had delayed his aim by a few minutes and that he would be late for his crucial meeting when we left around fifteen minutes later. He couldn't get any peace or relaxation for the rest of the trip and was always restless.

Goals, plans, and time control our lives in the West. Being busy is practically fashionable these days, and we frequently keep busy to avoid facing any potential concerns or anxieties we may have regarding love and intimacy. When was the last time you were too busy for love? Then, when you had some free time, you would quickly spend fifteen to twenty minutes before going to bed. Or perhaps it was a hasty morning activity before going to work.

Time has entered our lovemaking in this type of intercourse, bringing with it the pressure that something must happen, and quickly! We, therefore, gravitate toward orgasm because it feels nice in our haste to produce pleasure. Tantra, on the other hand, teaches us that making love requires time—lots and plenty of unhurried time. Hours must pass for sexual energy to unwind, bloom, and flower before it may provide the most fulfilling feelings of passionate love.

When we allow ourselves this chance, we discover wonderfully surprising and novel situations, where the energy itself celebrates in various ways every time. There is no way you could get bored. In actuality, we are the ones making the difference, as well as how much we can let go and embrace the present moment.

A healing force

When couples are at ease, open, and available to one another, perhaps newly in love or surrounded by stunning natural flora, this Tantric dimension opens up organically and unintentionally. Many of us have experienced this perfect moment where everything feels like heaven. I recall it happening to me on its own, late one night, in India, amid a heavy monsoon downpour. There was a sense of being engulfed in an intense whirlwind due to the thunder and severe rain. When time suddenly froze, my longtime partner and I were moving as one body, passionately and aimlessly, cognizant of our presence in the expanding present now, in his enormous bamboo bed. I have no idea how I got there; I was flying and glowing, ecstatically full of love for hours.

I may now deliberately and willfully enter this enigmatic present reality thanks to Tantra, rather than just by coincidence or accident. Many of our difficulties, worries, sadness, and even illnesses have a sexual component. We learn that sex is a spiritual energy that heals when we incorporate consciousness into sexuality as God and nature intended. Surprisingly, unlike what couples typically feel, sexual interest does not eventually fade. Contrastingly, the attraction grows stronger. As time goes on, the sexual experience becomes much more refined as the genitals develop a new level of ecstatic "intelligence" in their communication.

Tantra dispels the shadows and awakens the light, which is everyone's inheritance.

- Tensions of our sexual conditioning block our true orgasmic potential.

- Discover the journey of sex and forget about the end part.

- An unhurried approach creates a quality of timelessness, one of being present.

- Through this the sexual organs re-discover their ecstatic intelligence.

CHAPTER THREE

POLARITY AND THE POSITIVE POLES OF LOVE

THE BIGGEST INSIGHT OF TANTRA, in fact, its fundamental principle, is that male and female energies are complementary yet opposed powers. Similar to how yang and yin, dynamic and receptive, positive and negative, attract and complement one another (see fig. 4). This represents the idea that when men and women are united in a sexual union, their bodies' bio-energies interact to produce an ecstatic sexual experience. And all of this takes place passively. The Tantric path starts when we reconnect with and acknowledge our innate masculine and female polarity. Men and women must have opposing polarities or forces because this changes how we see the sex act.

Male and female polarities

Men and women are out of balance with one another as a result of our sexual indoctrination, which has tragically obscured our natural polarity. The bodies can be compared to two magnets with the ability to attract one other and form an attractive magnetic field. Our poles are covered in rust, dust, and fuzz, which obstructs the magnetic field and the passage of energy between them instead of being shining and dazzling to respond to each other vibrantly.

It almost seems as if we have upset the fundamental polarity or charge in our bodies by our programming pushing us toward orgasm. The male and female polarities are now hidden and covered by this cloud of disruption. To put it another way, the effort and activity we typically put into romantic relationships produce friction-style heat, or perhaps a screen of "over-charge" that is comparable to static electricity, which disrupts our genitals and prevents the sexual energy from responding through polarity.

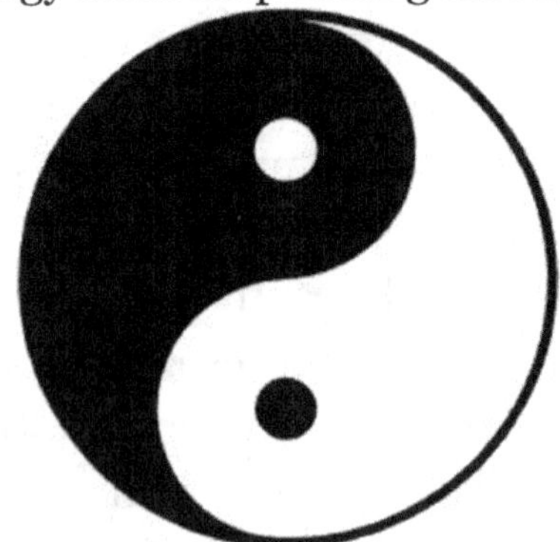

Fig. 4   Yin and Yang symbol of equal and opposite forces

We unknowingly fight against our blissful sexual potential when we make love by operating against the natural polarity of the sex organs. We can cleanse (decondition) ourselves of this energy disturbance by making conscious love, and the bodies will gradually and happily return to their natural male and female polarities. Guys start to feel more like themselves, and women start to feel more like themselves.

Because it has been our unhappy state for so long, we typically are not aware of this falsehood or disturbance in our polarity, but it is clear these days that ladies are becoming more tough and manly while a lot of men are becoming more macho, and violent. The sexual energy that is in distress is having negative consequences on both men and women. We were born with this imbalance, and until we are taught otherwise, as soon as we make love, we are perpetuating it.

Reeducating Ourselves About Sex

For ages, there has been very little direction around sex. When I ask my female clients how much information they received about their periods as girls, the response is often "none." Nothing at all to report. Many people received the necessary gear well in advance of the event, but that was it. For a woman, this is a monthly event that is intimately related to sex and childbirth, yet we rarely or never receive advice. What sexual knowledge do you possess as a parent that you could impart to your child? Most men and women have had zero exposure to this important area of their life. I found myself in a similar situation, and it took me some time and dedication to restore the sensitivity I had unknowingly lost. Instead of being focused on "doing" and going "there" toward orgasm, I had to learn how to unwind and "be here" when in a romantic relationship.

For me, accepting my polarity and watching myself sink deeper into it was a crucial first step. It surprised me to discover that my man was becoming more "positive," more dynamic, more vital, and more "here" as I worked on becoming more "negative" and passive, so to speak. I also focused on how to become more allowing, receptive, and conscious. This was not the same positive I had known in the past when falling in love might be characterized as a pressing intense linear event that produced a peak of energy.

That was virtually the complete opposite, similar to a peak inverting or bottoming out. It was something fresh and unique, extraordinarily joyous, circular, ecstatic, and deeply moving. Every time I reverted to my peak and release pattern, I had a sense of frustration, irritability, incompleteness, and distance from my partner.

I gradually understood that this new "style" of making love gave my life purpose—a spiritual aspect for which I had been looking in other places. I had the impression that I had been roaming through the desert for a while before finding a peaceful fireside. I gradually realized that love depended more on me and my consciousness than it did on him and that it was increased by an inner concentration rather than an exterior focus. In this way, everything was immediately put back in my control, and I realized that I was solely accountable for the standard of love in my life.

I became much more likable and loving when I made conscious love.

Loving In A Magnetic Field

Masculine and female energies are the positive and negative opposites of a single phenomenon, respectively. Each half by itself is insufficient; they can only coexist as a whole. But it's crucial to realize that any polarity, whether positive or negative, has its complementary opposing pole (see fig. 4). The essentially negative woman contains a balanced inner positive pole, and the primarily positive male also has an inner negative pole (an inner man).

In this sense, both are independent of one another and stand alone as a unit, each having a positive or negative internal attitude. Each body now can produce and transfer energy inside itself. The positive pole is located in the male body's genitalia, whereas the negative pole is located in the chest and heart region. The positive pole is located in the female's breasts and heart, while the negative pole is located in her genitalia, acting in natural opposition. A magnetic field is created between these positive and negative forces, allowing the sexual energy to flow and spiral upward through the body. The "rod of magnetism" (see fig. 5) is the name given to the magnetic field that exists between the two opposite poles.

A strong magnetic field is formed between these two "magnetic rods" when they are near one another. An "electrical" circuit is completed when they meet at their opposite poles while joined in a full-bodied sexual union.

The male sexual energy rises from the penis through the vagina to the woman's heart. Through the man's breasts, the feminine energy responds by entering his heart and traveling downhill to his sex core. The circulating bio-energies become a complete unit and can produce flickering light. Once the circuit is complete, electricity flows back and forth between the sexes in active and passive phases, with the sex changes occurring between the sexes. Tantra refers to this phenomenon as "the circle of light" since it is a divine bio-electricity that existed long before contemporary invention (see fig. 6). The utmost potential of man and woman as a spiritual force that may unlock the mysteries of life is represented by this potent polarity effect.

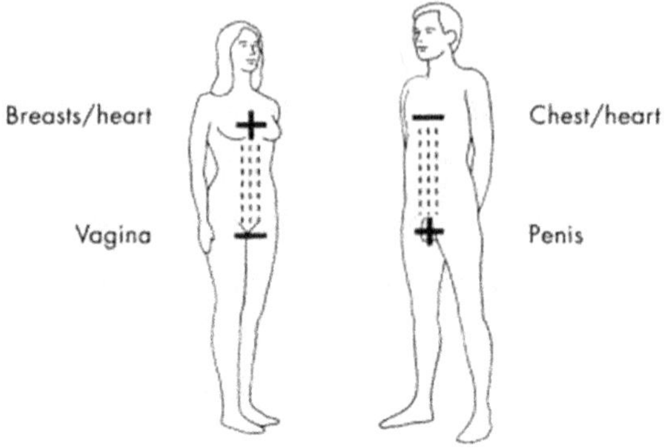

Fig. 5   Male and female bodies showing opposite polarities within and the rod of magnetism

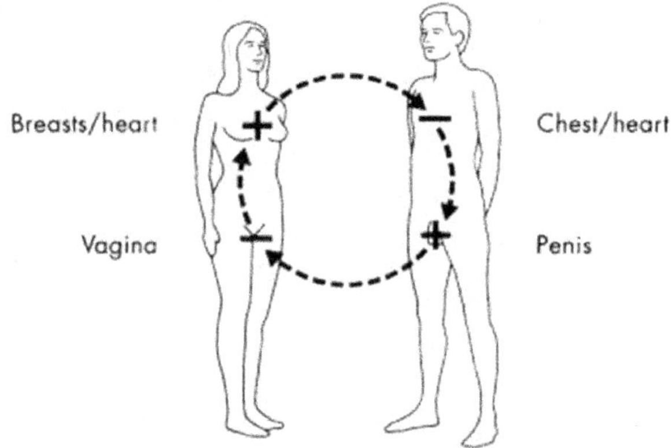

Fig. 6   Circular movement of energy between bodies creates a "circle of light"

In a very practical approach, we must incorporate this knowledge of polarity into our romantic endeavors. Since body energy moves from positive to negative, much like electricity, it is necessary to awaken the positive poles of the male and female bodies to start the deeper movement of sexual energy. The penis and breasts are referred to in Tantra as the "positive poles of love," which emphasizes the significance of this strategy. Every life originates from them; milk comes from women and semen from men. The level of sexual energy produced is greatly affected by how they are treated during foreplay and intercourse.

Generating sexual energy through polarity

In real terms, this indicates that a woman's breasts are incomparably more significant than her vagina. Yet, we often focus solely on both sexual organs during foreplay and lovemaking, which involves stroking and stimulation. We consider having sex as soon as feasible between these two, and typically, sex starts as soon as the guy has an erection and far before the woman is sexually awakened.

The penis is a man's positive and dynamic pole, and it is always ready. This is a woman's passive, negative, and receptive pole, which is not always ready. When we should be concentrating on the positive poles of love, the focus is accidentally directed toward the penis and the vagina, the organs of love. This strategy is quite popular, however, there is a significant misconception regarding female body energy, and this ignorance is the root of our profound dissatisfaction with sex.

Due to the inability to produce sexual energy through polarity, both men and women are extremely disappointed (if not outraged).

Even if it is exciting, foreplay that focuses on a woman's clitoris and vaginal region is energetically useless. She is unable to experience intense sexual arousal because her inner body polarity places less value on her genitalia. Her heart must be warmed, her breasts and nipples must be engaged, and she must welcome her bio-energy response, the positive pole. Warmth, receptivity, and willingness are spontaneously showered into the vagina by the love and energy that has been amassed here in the positive pole, awakening the passive pole.

The positive pole of love must be present before the organ of love can be prepared. When the male energy suddenly surges into the circuit upon penetration (or at any point thereafter), the vagina truly awakens, creating what might be defined as "electrical potential" between the penis and vagina. It is a unique sex experience. Before penetration, her breasts are given loving attention, which is crucial since it signals that she is physically and psychologically ready for intercourse. The lady will be perceived by the male as being with him, by his side, and moving in sync with him. He won't have to fight for his love, and neither will she have to try to offer it; there will just be a sense of oneness with a deep physiological yes from her. It is a real unity of the sexes.

This kind of polarity-based infatuation starts the process of creating a strong energy field between and within two bodies. The movement of the renowned serpent power—the kundalini energy, found at the base of the male spine—will be seen as a violent unfolding, jerking, ascending snake because the bio-electricity flowing inside this magnetic field follows a spiral pattern, which explains why.

Contrary to popular belief, the female kundalini energy source is located in the breasts rather than the spinal base. Energy cannot be raised from a negative core, which is why this is the case. This serpent will implode after a woman's breasts and heart have reached their full resonance, delicately unwinding and giving way from inside. Love can reach new heights with bio-electricity since the energy links and resonates deeply within the bodies and souls. Once the body's electricity takes over, a sensation of timelessness permeates, and each moment is joyful and orgasmic, something we may have only imagined, we can love intensely. As polarity has no beginning or end, only the potential for ever-increasing light, the pleasures of romantic love will develop.

The way to ecstatic sexual union

Returning to the inherent polarities where men become more macho and women more feminine, the art is in creating and harnessing duality. The ability to genuinely love and fulfill a woman in sex, which satisfies a man's greatest desire, causes him to feel more firmly planted, mature, responsible, loving, and energizing. There is genuine masculine authority and clarity. A woman starts to perceive herself as pure and sweet, the source of love and creation, and a delicate, scented femininity emerges as a result of receiving and giving this love. Harmony, mutual respect, and admiration are created when this inherent polarity is brought into balance. Love manifests as a tangible reality. As soon as we embrace polarity, an organic magnetic intelligence between the penis and vagina emerges. This intelligence grows stronger over time. The astonishing outcome is that making love becomes easier and easier for us as the body performs it on its own. The experience is, in fact, greater the less we do and the more we allow ourselves to be.

The penis, or lingham, is typically encircled by the vagina, or yoni, in the ancient Tantric symbol known as the Shivalingam, which is still widely used throughout India today. The yoni in this instance has a considerably deeper significance than only serving as a representation of the negative feminine pole, although being depicted in several intriguing shapes and patterns. Also, it serves as a conduit and a route to the heart via which the male positive, who serves as his counterpart, can connect with him. In a divine union, the positive male pole pierces the negative female pole, moves upward, and finally pierces the heart. When this occurs, the penis is beautifully enveloped and absorbed by the heart, creating a sort of golden interlocking effect. Ecstasy at its purest!

KEY POINTS:

- Male and female are attractive forces as are positive and negative.
- This polarity is the source of our sexual ecstasy.
- Each body carries the opposite pole within which forms a "magnetic rod".
- Two bodies in union create a powerful magnetic field and circulate bio-energy.
- To activate the sex energy a woman's breasts must be loved and caressed.

CHAPTER FOUR

AWARENESS OF BODY AND MIND

The combination of sexual activity and meditation is THE ART OF TANTRA, to put it simply. It is a simultaneous physical and spiritual occurrence in which two seemingly incompatible extremes merge to form one. When this occurs, a magical quality emerges, and we get the impression that we're entering a fourth dimension where the "present now," which has been enveloping us in mystery, awakens. Everything in this realm sparkles and glows, bringing a newfound appreciation for our surroundings, our lover, and ourselves as well as freshness to the eyes and a song of love to the heart. When the vital energy of the universe, which pulses with life itself, is passing through us, we feel incredibly porous and sensitive.

We don't experience this sensitivity or aliveness in traditional sex since we typically aren't attentive or conscious of what is happening. While we may think we are having fun, we are usually only going through the motions, frequently automatically, or regularly. By endeavoring to be mindful of what is happening in each instant during conscious sex, we create the possibility of having a richer feeling of love each time. This occurs as a result of our understanding of the true nature of sexual energy; this understanding turns sex into love.

A natural meditation

Tantra encourages us to become awake and conscious of ourselves as we make love because of this. Our focus is within, we are present to our senses and emotions, and we are "here," so we don't lose our way or become robotic. Meditation naturally develops when having sex. Most people think of meditation as being done in a solitary, upright, still, and motionless state, however, this is simply one type of meditation. Sexual movement doesn't have to be frantic; it can be calm.

As in ballet, tai chi, or swimming, they can be centered around a stillness. Contrary to common assumption, sex acts are the most conducive to the emergence of meditation because their intense physical pleasure draws us, sometimes even compels us, into the awareness of what is happening at the time. The perception of "here," or "being here," that results from this knowledge of the current situation give birth to a sense of inner calm and tranquility. This is the coveted result of meditation. There is silence, depth, and presence only by bringing consciousness to reside within the body, whether we are moving or still. The consciousness is unmoving, unchanging, and tranquil throughout all of the body's movement, position changes, and even flight.

We can start to experience consciousness by slowing down and being relaxed during sex to perceive the present. We must take the time to hear and pay close attention to subtleties that emerge from inner calm or focus. A new degree of sensuous perception and sensitivity develops over time and with familiarity as a couple continues to enjoy their intimate encounters in this unhurried manner. The sensation grows more exhilarating and enjoyable. In this way, having sex can develop into an intense continuing meditation in which the bodies and spirits of two individuals come into communion.

We discover that awareness is at the heart of the conversation when we talk about altering the way we make love. It is a vital component in elevating sex to a new level. As we make love, we must continuously pay attention to our bodies and become aware of exactly what we are doing and feeling. This is the first step in becoming more aware. Slowly, slowly, we start to pay attention to every gesture, movement, and breath. When we develop the ability to observe and be with all that occurs inside of our bodies, the act of having sex itself comes to dominate our attention and awareness. And the simple act of experiencing it and witnessing it changes it.

We will be startled to discover that our bodies are a world unto themselves with several realities working at once when we bring awareness to them. The body experiences specific vibrations, tingling, warmth, and even light as the heart beats and the breath rises and falls. If our brains are obsessed with something or someone else, such as forms outside of ourselves, their colors, contents, or characters, our awareness will become scattered and ineffectual. Our desire for orgasm also significantly reduces our consciousness since we overlook the current moment when we are focused on an impending occurrence. We are absent, even if we are one second ahead of ourselves. We must start creating a presence in the place of our tendency of being absent in sex as we start to confront it. It takes a great deal of mindfulness to stay in the body and the present moment.

Focus on the present moment

Sex gives us the chance to work on and sharpen our consciousness so that we may genuinely create the current moment. In sex, we learn to "be" more and "do" less. The beautiful Tantric experience results from this. When there is no overarching objective, the life force suddenly bursts forth in a spontaneous and unrestrained manner. Because of how powerful and vibrant the natural affinity between the penis and vagina is, it makes it simple to be in the moment.

For example, when we walk, the sensation of our feet making touch with the ground through our shoes is not particularly acute (although it can be if you want it to be). In the same way, using a wooden spoon while cooking does neither excite nor excite us greatly. The mind might easily wander to unrelated topics. Unlike when we are walking, cooking, or doing any other routine work, sexual union's intensity and profoundly engrossing nature make it simpler for us to be conscious of the illusive present now. The pleasures of sex combined with awareness create an encounter whose very nature might bring us back to the present.

Be aware of yourself

Tantra demands that we focus our mind and concentration on ourselves to help us into the present now. I've discovered that in traditional sex, the focus is typically on the partner first and foremost as we concentrate on his or her pleasure. What's his condition? I would ponder this. Is he feeling well? Do I have this right? Is this a good or bad amount? Nearly more significant than I was was he. I became aware that I didn't feel rooted below or like I had a strong inner connection to my body when I focused on my partner in these and other ways. I was dressed to the nines and making out with someone else.

Tantra taught me to turn my focus inward, to stop thinking about the man, and to start by interacting with my energy. It taught me to make love to myself first before worrying about him, to bring consciousness inward, lower, and back into my body, and to feel my tummy and my breath. Although it may seem absurd, this is the key! It fosters a state of ease and relaxation where natural intimacy and attraction develop and uncertainties are more easily overcome.

It indicates that before I attach one body to another, I must first energize and unite with my own. I present my body to my partner, attuned inside, vibrant and joyful, and prepared for a passionate embrace. This mindset of putting yourself first, grounding and centering yourself within, allows for so much more to occur in love.

Initially, this was made clear to me when I was performing and instructing bodywork. I've spent the majority of my life enjoying giving massages to people. To my dismay, I discovered that the spirit and joy of giving vanished when I focused on a specific result. I had decided that I needed to be more qualified, so I learned some new, sophisticated, and advanced techniques. After some time, I decided to give up any elaborate techniques I had acquired and go back to the greasy simplicity of massage, gliding along the musculature and cruising along the body's contours.

When looking for knots and tough sinewy pieces, I felt the wonderful textures, each of which had a captivating narrative of its own. They were always the "juiciest" locations for me to experiment with, and I soon stopped paying attention to my technique. Instead, I started to concentrate solely on the surface I was touching. How did the tissues of your body feel underneath? The fingertips most enjoyed searching in what way? What would make me feel the tastiest if I were resting here? Where and how did my hands desire to touch the most?

I started to lose interest in the person I was massaging and started to focus solely on my body movements, breathing, internal relaxation, and the area of the body beneath my scouring hands. I discovered that the more I concentrated on my hands and body, the more the individual appeared to relax and the more the body would emit an almost ringing silence. They would feel incredibly rejuvenated, deeply rested, at peace, and well benefit from the massage. Time had no meaning to them; an hour of bodyless eternity had passed. The ability of the other person to relax back into themselves increased as I became more preoccupied with myself and the present. The people always felt better, sometimes even richer, whenever I simply loved touching their bodies during a session instead of thinking about their physical issues. I recall feeling guilty when I did this. Today, I advise my massage students to put their attention on themselves and the pure joy of touching and giving rather than worrying about their technique and instead just infuse their touch with love and consciousness. The individual employing the technique is more valuable than the technique itself.

Relax into your body

Similarly to this, to make love, we need to take back control, focus on and get comfortable with the inside of our bodies, and learn to relax all over. Your lover is more relaxed when you are relaxed, and vice versa. The present moment becomes more important to us when we unwind, and as a result, sexual experience may naturally arise. The intensity of focusing the mind on the delicateness of the genitalia during sexual union stimulates the body's consciousness to awaken. Sex then turns into a form of divine meditation and the body into a temple.

I advise couples to forget about each other, their personalities, or their difficulties and concentrate on their inner world because our new strategy is fundamentally a change from mind to body. This method helped me when I was retraining myself since it let my thoughts fade into the background while using my body as an anchor to establish my inner reality. We must learn to broaden our sensory awareness, including its sensations and perceptions, because the senses and sensuality are substantially improved via awareness and because love is created in the physical body.

What is going on inside our bodies? Then where? Keep in mind that you must shift your emphasis from the periphery to the center, from the mind's external focus to the body's internal focus. What and where am I feeling right now? How does it feel in reality? Where exactly in my body am I experiencing the rebirth of life?

In this room, where is the light? At the start of a class, I frequently advise couples to search inside themselves "for a spot that feels like home, a root."

If you come upon such a place, stay there and rest. Give it some color or light, then imagine expanding it. See it as a place in your body where you can anchor yourself and find some tranquility. It might be anywhere—the stomach, the heart, the genitalia, the lower back—but not the head! Hold it in your awareness wherever it is and learn to live in its sensation. Do not forget that you may always go back inside if you discover that you have unintentionally left the house, which will happen frequently.

We must always take a step back into our interior area and exit the exterior space. It seems as though we must physically enter our bodies to build the inside space and keep growing it. People's inside spaces must be "forced" to expand because the outside area is typically larger than the inside space.

It seems as though the gap between the bodies that usually divides them genuinely comes alive, like a magnetic field, when each person first devotes time and attention to his or her own body by widening their internal space. You become conscious of the life emanating from your own body, which allows you to communicate with your lover's presence and body via the air between you.

The body's inner awareness or sense is a far more sensitive phenomenon than the mind. It is challenging to reach down into the immensity of the body and perceive what is specifically occurring there while our attention is preoccupied with thought. It's challenging to "be" in the body. One contributing aspect is that we move our bodies into physical touch far too quickly when we first start making love. To make the other feel good, we condense what might otherwise be a lengthy and lovely discussion into a matter of seconds.

Each person is dragged away from their home, out of consciousness, and off-center as a result of this. We put more effort into doing something to the other, such as rubbing, touching, or caring for them, as opposed to feeling oneself by dropping inside and absorbing the other, being pleasant and uncomplicated. We have lost touch with who we are as people and have turned into human "doings."

Let your body be your guide

To experiment with this approach, try this exercise:

Lay on your sides with your bodies slightly apart and facing each other in bed before initiating a sexual relationship. Distract your attention from your companion and place it on your own body. For a few seconds, close your eyes and feel your awareness shifting from the outside to the inside. You can visualize yourself moving vertebrae by vertebrae down your spine, down the back, down into the pelvis, and connecting with the energy in the legs and the base of your body. Give yourself some time and persevere for a while. Before you combine your bodies, this revitalizes your own body. Open your eyes and stare at one another after a while.

You remain conscious of your own body throughout this. Breathe. Let your jaw drop. After a short while, steadily get closer to your lover while maintaining your inner attention. Start with a meeting of the fingertips and ease into an embrace; the slower the better. Let it be more of a "happening" than a "doing." Keep a keen awareness of the warmth and texture of each area of your body as it touches and envelops the other. You will ultimately notice that the bodies are drawn or sucked together, attracted like magnets, if you wait long enough just "being."

Let go of your intentions and just enjoy becoming closer to the one you love. Our awareness of ourselves and our lover is significantly increased as we enter into love with this gradual sensitivity. This sluggish, lackadaisical approach has a vibrant reaction from bodily energies as well.

You can do this as well when you are reuniting with someone after being apart. Before giving a hug, pause, remain still, and take a few seconds to focus within and anchor yourself in your body, your legs, and your feet. Next, take a modest step forward and ease into a progressive hug with your partner. Maintain your calm, let your shoulders fall, avoid exerting too much physical effort, and breathe. Be in the body with awareness, let the bodies greet one another, and allow them to melt into one another.

This method of drawing the awareness inward as opposed to projecting it forth makes the body's internal environment more delicate. Your attention was diverted, so you become conscious of things you were previously unaware of as having sensation or sensitivity. Yet while we are having a romantic relationship, ideas of climax regularly take up our minds. Your dimensionality—that magnificent interior between your front and back that explodes into sensitivity like an inner fireworks display—begins to become apparent when you can be present in your body.

Switch off your mind

By shifting our attention from our outer manifestation to our inner impression, or from an outward expression to an inside impression, we increase our body's sensitivity. Tantra brings us back to sexuality and sex. Due to the mind's integration with the sex act, we now experience our sexuality rather than the genuine force of sex. We must begin by turning off or disassociating from the thinking portion of ourselves to return to the pure and natural condition of sex.

The mind's amazing capacity for fantasizing may be the largest distraction in modern sex. Many people's sex lives now revolve around sexual fantasy. We frequently engage in sexual fantasies when making love while being unaware of the moment. Instead of focusing on the current companion, we are imagining a different one or a different scenario. As a result, we are not experiencing the body as it is. Instead, the body is being propelled or motivated by the mind's use of fiction. Sexual fantasies can become routine as if we were continually running the same script.

I'm confident that almost all of us have utilized sexual imagery—real or imagined—to arouse and sustain interest in the sex act. Most of the time, we employ sexual fantasies to spur us on to orgasm since they enable us to achieve heights. It performs amazingly well! For the mind to deliver such tremendous, even instantaneous outcomes, it must be declared to be a powerful tool. But, sexual imagination is a terrific diversion since it takes our attention away from the present moment and the person we are making love with.

Tantra accepts this creative capacity of the mind in its wisdom. It promotes its rerouting into the body. Instead, the power of the mind can be used to activate healthy energy flow throughout the body. And this occurs as a result of the fact that energy eventually follows imagination. We've all given it a go, so we know it works. Hence, rather than being a source of distraction during sex, imagination can be a useful tool.

For instance, if we start to visualize circles of light and energy flowing through our bodies, energetic connections between the positive and negative poles (within and outside of yourself), energy flowing from a man into a woman, a woman absorbing this golden light, energy radiating from the heart and breasts, or energy leaping from the penis, we will eventually start to feel as though this is what is happening. The energy can be visualized as a flowing stream of golden light or as lightning or even as lightning that jumps and leaps. This may be simpler for men to use.

A return to innocence

Although it may be vague at first, your awareness will assist in fanning it, which causes energy to build and expand. Some people are better able to "sense energy" than others. Please utilize your imagination if it is difficult for you; it will do wonders for the body. The use of your imagination can enhance any experiences in which you feel the energy moving within you. In this way, the inner energy circuits—which get more and more dynamic with time—are guided by the mind.

We must constantly remind ourselves that the first stage in the shift from sexuality to sex—the return of sex to the innocence of the body—is to be aware of the inner song of the body, and the second step is to be conscious of the thoughts. Even when we are not using fantasy in the sex act, we frequently have all kinds of potentially harmful thoughts running through our heads. It is surprising to learn what else is going on inside of us once we become aware of our thoughts, which are believed to number 50,000 every day. When the kind of lovemaking I had dreamed of was occurring in my early sexual life, I discovered to my horror that I would often find myself daydreaming and thinking about other things. I couldn't believe it could be anything so simple as where to eat dinner! I had trouble getting absorbed in sex. Since then, I've learned that sexual energy is so delicate and nuanced that even a fleeting thought can disrupt its normal magnetic flow.

A gradual process

It is not as if we have to stop thinking when we are bringing our mental process to conscious awareness. We cannot! The issue is that we do think! Though there is little we can directly do to influence thinking, there are indirect ways we might approach it. The important thing is to become aware of the thoughts, which are running through your head. By becoming aware of them, you are brought back into the present and the thread connecting them is severed. You dissociate or "cur with the mind" only by admitting that you were thinking. Once you've had enough, you come back to the present. Instead of starting an internal dialogue criticizing yourself for being absent and non-present, just swiftly return to the present. Until you find yourself back in the cognitive process, stay present and focused on the physicality and sensuality of consciousness in the body.

After you become aware, return to your body without delay.

The miracle of the phenomena of consciousness is that all that is required of you is for you to become aware. A change can be made by just observing your thoughts and becoming conscious of the physical patterns they cause. As if a bridge is built, the mind becomes more at ease, content, and tuned in to the body. It's crucial to keep in mind that the Tantrie journey is a gradual one when couples set out on it. It is a change in consciousness rather than a technique or an abrupt transformation. You must be it because you cannot do it. The process of developing calm is ongoing and takes time. If you don't expect large changes or quick outcomes, it will help. It doesn't always work out that way. True change is made up of innumerable, occasionally imperceptible, little adjustments that are ingrained in the body. Take note of the little, less noticeable things that occur to you, including how they make you feel, where you feel it, and where the delight comes from. As a result of the consciousness that the sexual act brings to the body, it starts to change and develop into a source of love that benefits the body, mind, and soul.

- Awareness of mind and body transforms the sexual experience into love.
- Shift the awareness from outside to inside.
- This focus creates a "root" within the body.
- Challenge thinking by consciously experiencing bodily sensations.
- Use power of imagination to amplify and expand energy movement.

CHAPTER FIVE

PENETRATING INNOCENCE: THE LOVE KEYS

When we engage in CONVENTIONAL SEX, we might compare our bodies to an open flower with petals that are reaching out into the world. When we are all concentrating on one another, the energy is predominantly directed away from the center.

Learning to live through the body

Tantra involves deliberately inverting the blossom; the petals are drawn back into the core and inverted toward it as if going back to becoming a bud. Most of the energy is directed into our center. The Love Keys force us to turn inward and concentrate on our inner selves, which we must consciously expand. The Love Keys assist in bringing our awareness from the edges to the center, allowing us to concentrate our awareness within the body.

We can stay more and more in the present moment by grounding awareness in the body and using the body as a constant reference point. The body is the only thing that truly exists right now, thus increasing our chances of being happy overall requires learning to live through the body. We choose the straightforward pleasure of the flesh, which is a gift from God, over the confused, troubled, and wandering mind.

If we make love knowingly, especially if we make love consciously repeatedly, polarity, the central idea of Tantra that the genitals produce an energy of their own, starts to arise on its own. The Love Keys will use the knowledge of polarity and the significance of interacting with the positive poles (which might be called the background Love Key) to transform the body into a means, an anchor, and a bridge to keep us firmly planted in the sexual present. The Love Keys will direct us to numerous body locations that provide access points to being "here and now" in the present.

These Love Keys have helped me countless times, and as I sank into them, layer by layer, I was gradually able to ground my awareness in my own body and reclaim my confidence in myself. Old sexual scars were able to leave the body, repressed energy was released, and I was able to change to a higher frequency as a result of bringing consciousness into the act. When residing in India, I first offered the Love Keys to my experimental group of Westerners and was astounded by the remarkably quick response. Both men and women had sparkling eyes, and love was in the air! In a matter of days, I was able to unravel and rearrange in myself what had taken me years to do. It was miraculous.

This gave me comfort because it showed that our bodies react similarly out of instinct. Since then, I've found that regardless of whether a couple has been together for one night or 32 years, or if they are in their teens or their sixties, the response is the same. Love grows when we are conscious. However, it is important to emphasize that creating "the present" with the Love Keys and in the body is a continuous process. It never does.

Although there may initially be a sense of enchantment and a more laid-back approach to sex, it takes time for the sexual present to become deeply ingrained in the body. You can't expect to be operating in one manner for many years, preoccupied with fantasies or the sexual high of orgasm, and then all of a sudden switch to a completely different way of being.

Moving Away From Old Patterns

A couple must understand that making love is an art, a process, and not an immediate affair. It is composed of little movements that may have enormous effects. But the more we use the Love Keys, the more we may practice breaking free from our ingrained habits and entering the experience of the here and now. It involves continually going back to the body. We occasionally succeed and occasionally fail. Sometimes we will become engrossed in the need for orgasm; if this happens, please indulge and fully enjoy it. At the same time, be conscious of the fact that we are selecting this to be what is happening.

This is a fantastic first step. It makes us more aware of the activity we are engaging in, and with time and practice, when we can stay in the body while making love, no longer pushed to do but glad to be, the body regains its innate sensitivity and consciousness.

Your relationship with your partner will improve thanks to The Love Keys, and a new level of intimacy will develop. A strong foundation for love will be created, much like learning a new language. You may unwind and take more time to concentrate on what is happening inside your body, especially between the penis and vagina, thanks to the awareness cultivated by the Love Keys. Positive and negative poles start responding to one another and vibrating beautifully as the genitals' sensitivity rises and polarity eventually takes hold. Sexual activity ceases to involve the mind and returns to the physical body.

Take The Time To Create Stillness

But, this will take time. It could be difficult to feel anything at all when you first try a new manner of experiencing the genitals. Even attempting to feel could be an effort. We have always relied on a lot of friction for our sexual experience up to this moment, but now we are looking for a sensitivity that lies behind this surface-level sensation. A finer, more brilliant, and gratifying layer is coming into contact with you.

Moreover, even though you will always be able to feel excited, you are getting past the first intensity and overwhelming aspect of this excitement. On the verge of stepping underneath it. You must become more relaxed physically and mentally to feel something that was previously only faintly perceptible. It takes time and dedication to reach this level of sensitivity, but the payoff is enormous.

You will feel open, vulnerable, and even a little unsteady when you first start utilizing the Love Keys. You are breaking through your innocence, therefore this is only normal. Like starting to make love for the first time, it is as though going back to that pure, childish state of being present and playful. A variety of colors make up the new scene. It's acceptable to laugh if you feel awkward, humiliated, or slightly stupid. I have had many fits of unrestrained, loud laughter, and each time I did, I immediately felt better, more alive, and at ease. Allow your tears to fall when you're upset, accept them, and don't hold them back. Intimacy and fulfilling lovemaking require you to relax into a deeper, more true layer of yourself, which can only be achieved by the expression of suppressed inner tensions such as laughter and tears.

We should be real and lighthearted in this sort of play. Between these two, there lies a world. Sincerity is a feeling that comes from the heart, whereas seriousness comes from the mind. Seriousness enjoys a tried-and-true recipe, while sincerity prefers to experiment and learn. It's similar to peeling an onion to play with the Love Keys. To fully experience the glory of relaxation in the body, one must always peel back another layer and take another step.

Love can profoundly into you when you and your partner are allowed to be loose and explore with each other, playfully and willingly with commitment. You will soon discover that love is not some untamed wind sweeping through and over you beyond your conscious control, but something that you can create via your consciousness, that love is in your very own hands.

Explore And Experiment

To experiment with sex, we require an open mind and a loving mentality. We as a couple must be willing to challenge our ingrained patterns of romantic behavior, which means we may have to give up things we have previously really valued. We will need to support one another in breaking or releasing the mechanical or doing aspects of sex since for the majority of us, it has become a relatively mechanical orgasm-hunting experience. People will frequently admit that the excitement of it is similar to an addiction. But, it will be challenging to appreciate what we are getting if we continue to concentrate on the typical benefits of sex and what we are giving up.

We need the patience and willingness to let go of the old ways, as well as a humorous, sincere approach to get ready for the new because there is frequently a lag between letting go and gaining. It is most beneficial when both parties adopt similar views since this commitment to exploration and the unexpected makes ultimate cooperation and discovery feasible.

For instance, it could be difficult to remain open to exploration when experiencing intense sexual heat and passion. You can suddenly feel an intense urge to have an orgasm. And right now, nothing feels more crucial!

However, if your partner can assist you in returning to the present moment, suddenly the opportunity for you to unwind arises. By making the enormous decision to give in to this compulsive urge, the mystery of sex will start to reveal itself to you. To develop your love and clarify your sexual experience, you must have your partner's support and awareness. When couples cooperatively make love, they support one another and learn from one another as well as through one another.

Together, they find the route to sex relaxation. Alone, it is not feasible. Stepping away from our unconscious sexual qualities becomes all but impossible when one partner consistently opposes the efforts of the other. It will be quite difficult to explore new territory without mutual willingness.

Even if you have undoubtedly made love thousands of times, there must be an attitude of vulnerability from the beginning, a humble admission that neither of you knows anything about making love. When introducing herself, a woman I worked with said she had at least 3,500 times made love in the same way and was here to see what else was possible. A lack of vulnerability may result from one or both partners' unwillingness to challenge established sexual routines and venture into uncharted territory.

If you believe that you understand what it takes to make love and how this enigmatic energy functions, there won't be room for other, perhaps more complex and lasting experiences. Instead, you must be prepared to name all of your emotions as well as your sex-related anxieties and doubts. The greater orgasmic potential of sex cannot be realized if your thinking is too rigid.

Banish rules from the bedroom

We must keep in mind that there are no guidelines for making love. It is more a matter of awareness when using the Love Keys. While we can learn and grow via awareness and teaching ourselves, rules are imposed on us and eventually entail disobedience. Making concepts stiff and immovable is a mind-defeating propensity, especially when we feel uneasy about not knowing what might come next. It is not the same as figuring things out for yourself through experimentation if you have to do it. "It works for me," as opposed to "I must," is different. A woman finds it very simple to become rule-oriented because she is typically the partner who makes fewer physical displays, making doing less work at first. Instead of acknowledging her fragility in the situation, I have all too frequently witnessed women enforcing rules and verbally condemning their partners. The male will respond by rebelling or ceasing to cooperate because he feels reprimanded and that his ego is being endangered.

Tantra offers ideas rather than rules when fears manifest in a novel sexual form. We can tell ourselves, "Do this," and when we do, we obtain practical experience that enables us to develop new rules and orientations. We are two people working as a team like scientists slicing through millennia of misunderstandings with their voracious curiosity. The ways of Tantra are those of patience, love, respect, and understanding.

Choosing Which Love Keys To Try

The nine broad categories of Eyes, Breath, Communication, Genital Awareness, Touch, Relaxation, Gentle Penetration, Deep Penetration, and Rotating Positions are used to group the Love Keys in Part 2. Each of the Love Keys helps us use our bodies to enter the present moment. There are keys within keys, as you will discover as you read each of the various Love Keys. Each Love Key offers a variety of doable advice that can be applied to romantic activities right away.

There is a lot to take in, so try not to use all the Love Keys at once and become stressed. As you read, observe which keys you respond to, which feel natural, and which pique your interest. Afterward, begin with these. You can start adding additional ones as soon as you start to feel secure in each of these. Also, after some trial-and-error, it's likely to make more sense, you'll comprehend more, or you'll develop an interest in things that had before piqued none of your interest.

It's a special dance, a trip, and an adventure. Your experience and perception will both deepen as you experiment. You are likely to notice a qualitative shift in your lovemaking even if you only adopt two Love Keys at first, such as keeping eye contact and taking slow, deep breaths. You are free to pick what you want to embrace; you do not have to.

Also, it is a lengthy process because a shift in consciousness, rather than a dramatic alteration, is taking place.

A year after their first session, I recall a couple telling me that after much experimentation with the Love Keys, they continued to enjoy the orgasms. They were able to be more loving and present thanks to the Love Keys, which was wonderful. To top it all off, they would experience an orgasm that resembled a small amount of whipped cream.

They carried on their investigation while participating in an additional workshop. Then, over the phone, after 2.5 years since our first conversation, the woman said, "You know, none of us is any longer interested in an orgasm! It's astounding considering how significant it once was. But now that we've slowly figured out how to stay here, it's a lot nicer and more enjoyable, so why bother with orgasms? And we are so in love and happy."

The beauty is that once consciousness is introduced to the act of sexuality, a process is launched and the old routines or patterns gradually leave the system. Consciousness grows and encounters new things. Therefore don't be scared to experiment with some of the Love Keys while you are making love. Simply give one or two a try and see the results. If you and your partner decide to experiment, you can select which you should do first. The influence on sexual energy can frequently be amplified when both lovers are utilizing the same Love Keys, such as combining positive poles and breathing, but this is not necessary.

Even if you don't plan or don't have a committed partner with whom to experiment, you can find yourself feeling suddenly inspired or ready to try something out. You might be surprised. When I told a friend in a workshop that the Love Key relaxation also included relaxing the vaginal muscles, she wasn't entirely convinced. She kept quiet at the time, but when she was later playing with her lover, she recalled this advice and consciously released her vagina after telling herself, "Okay, let it go!" The penis instantly dove into the recesses of the vagina as it enlarged and opened, pushing and probing upward while appearing almost appreciative.

Spread the awareness throughout your entire body when you select a certain Love Key to experiment with. For instance, if you decide to concentrate on your positive pole, avoid being overly preoccupied with it. Don't let it overshadow everything else so that it creates tension in your body rather than allowing your body to dissolve into calm. Relax your mind by visualizing it opening wide and fanning out if you notice that you are thinking about something too much. Sweep your awareness over the entire body, from top to bottom and back again, fusing the parts with the whole. As a result, the sexual energy spreads and grows, uniting the body as an organic whole.

How The Love Keys Will Help You Change Your Relationship For The Better

Tantra offers three suggestions for how we might explore our sexuality to effectively purge or de-condition ourselves of unconscious sexual practices that negatively impact the quality of the love in our lives and help us remove the harsh layer of our uncaring, uninformed past. You'll get help with this from the Love Keys. The first step is to break the habit of having orgasms. But take note of the fact that when we do go for it, we are essentially absent and ahead and so comparatively unconscious.

The second is to switch from engaging in sex and being involved. Furthermore take note of the fact that, while not being interested in the climax, we nonetheless feel compelled to take action to engage in a sexual encounter. The third involves relaxing and being mindful of the current moment to reclaim our original genital sensitivity (magnetic intelligence). This procedure depends on one another. The easier it is to rebuild genital sensitivity, the more you confront your tendencies. It is simpler to alter your routines the more awareness you give to your innate intellect. You might concentrate on one component on some days, another on others, and all of them together on other days. Making love, as opposed to merely comprehending it intellectually, is the only way for sex to undergo a complete re-education. The discipline of letting go of the sexual energy and learning to "be" results in the demotivation of many ingrained emotional patterns, compulsions, responses, and issues. Gradually, the silver thread of consciousness that weaves throughout the body retraces the surge into oblivion and the energy it uses.

KEY POINTS:

- The Love Keys strengthen rapport with your lover.

- Curiosity and the spirit of cooperation are vital keys to exploration.

- Expand your "inside space" through immediate bodily sensitivity.

- Let your experience teach and guide you.

- A shift in consciousness is a gradual process of unveiling sexual ecstasy.

CHAPTER SIX

THE EYES

THE EYES ARE INCREDIBLY DESIRABLE. You will frequently experience a surge of sex when two people look each other in the eyes. If you've ever had the chance to lay next to your lover and just look at each other, it may be a huge turn-on and a crucial component of foreplay. This is due to the fact that the eyes are strong sexual energy pathways. They expose us to the realities of the present moment and expose our innocence and nakedness. This enables us to be genuine. We can see where we are and who we are with when our eyes are open.

The sexual encounter with your partner becomes more vibrant and dynamic when this route through the eyes is opened. It is known that when we stare out through our eyes for regular vision, 80% of our energy is projected, discharged, and thrown out. Those with a structural misalignment, where the head and ears are awkwardly placed much ahead of the shoulders, are easily identifiable as having this strain. But, because our eyes are built to receive images, we can see without exerting any effort. Yet, it occurs. The image is taken in by the eye.

This suggests that when we look, we lose a lot of energy from the eyes. That happens every day as we constantly scan our surroundings, keeping an eye on what is going on, looking for amusing diversion, some novelty someplace, and trying to stay one step ahead of ourselves. While there is absolutely no connection at all between our eyesight and the inner dimensions of the body, our eyes are more closely tied to the mind and its restlessness.

Making and keeping eye contact

Similarly, when making love. I remember being so anxious and embarrassed that I laughed when I first started to keep my eyes open and look directly into my lover's eyes. I felt so totally unnatural. With the painful realization that I had never genuinely been "here" before, sincere before, I could have easily started crying. I was used to making love either with my eyes closed or in the dark, so I wasn't truly present for my partner right then and there. Yet after a short period of experimentation, I became used to it, and opening my eyes quickly evolved into a crucial energetic link between myself and my partner. I felt oddly lacking without it.

In our culture, it's common to feel uncomfortable looking someone in the eyes. We glance at each other's mouths, their shoes, their hair, the baby, and away while we talk to one another. We hardly ever lock gaze for more than a few seconds at a time. Eye contact is sometimes even perceived as an intrusion, a violation of our privacy, or a challenge to our authority.

I urge you to persevere even if maintaining eye contact while making love initially feels awkward because there is so much to gain from doing so. You will frequently experience an instantaneous sexual response within you, and it is the most amazing sharing of energy. By identifying the personality masks I wear, eye contact has also enabled me to develop presence in my lovemaking. I felt a freshness and it appeared there was less haze obscuring the scene around me after I had laughed and sobbed my way through them. A feeling of closeness and natural intimacy developed, and the loneliness vanished. Eventually, as my relaxation grew deeper, I tried to receive my partner through my eyes, taking him inside of my body.

I closed my eyes and looked deeply down into my body with my inner eye whenever I felt that my open eyes were obstructing the consciousness in my vagina.

Seeing and being seen

Eye contact is an art form in and of itself. I found it helpful to start by letting my eyes experience what is referred to as "soft vision." This indicates that I was receptive and let everything into my eyes. Normal vision involves us looking from the inside out, but you may deliberately reverse this occurrence and attempt looking from the outside in, as if the world were seeing through your own eyes. They are merely present and open, receiving, like windows. Through the window, sunshine streams into the space. Via your eyes and body, the outside world enters you. As you open up your eyes to everything in your field of vision, they become responsive, gentle, and welcoming.

When your lover and you lock eyes and gaze at one other tenderly, you are allowing yourself to be seen. You are here, making love to your spouse, firmly planted in the experience thanks to this contact and the awareness of the immediacy.

There is an easy method for doing this on your own. Visit a park and observe a tree. Look at it closely rather than just passing by. Enjoy the green, the leaves, and the life. Now close your eyes and take some time to unwind. Open your eyes once more, and this time, imagine that the tree is looking at you instead of you at it. Invite the tree into you through your eyes. See how much of the green livingness you can let permeate you. Take it inside your body's cells. Try it next with a cloudy, clear sky, or a stunning sunset. Give nature permission to peek inside of you and to pierce you. See how this technique heightens your awareness, blurs your boundaries, and makes you feel more a part of the environment.

Now that the room is sufficiently lit to see, take a delicate look into your partner's eyes. Pick the eye that seems most comfortable and natural to you. Let yourself simply "be" and be observed. With your eyes, take in the energy, allowing it to enter your body. Through your eyes, invite your partner inside of you. In reality, you are receiving your own energy's backflow, which fills and enlarges your heart while it is inverted and falls back on it. Moreover, the third eye picks it up. Spend some time now on the other eye. Take note of the differences between the right and left eyes, including their various hues and patterns. Which eye is more difficult for you? Just which is softer? Which one triggers your sexual desire? Spend some time with each eye and get used to being at ease with both of them. Avoid quickly switching between one eye and the other. This might make your partner uncomfortable. That may occur if one of you is anxious, so try to assist each other decompress by giving each other a gentle stroke or caress. It is very normal to be uncertain at this time. Try your best to let any pressure you may be feeling out. Give each other a moment to relax by closing your eyes and taking a few deep breaths.

It's crucial to avoid staring at the other person since doing so fosters a sensation of strangeness and distance rather than one of proximity or contact. Instead of scrutinizing someone, the goal should be to let them in and allow yourself to be seen. You are only employing your will when you stare; there is nothing behind your eyes. Be natural, be you, and blink. Do not exert yourself excessively by believing that you must always be vigilant. When your body is positioned so that your lover's eyes are not within easy reach of your own, you can even find it impossible to keep your eyes open.

Close your eyes if you need to

Make eye contact when you can, and avoid it when you can't as a general rule. Sometimes you need to close your eyes and feel exactly what is going on inside your body to re-focus yourself and find your core. The key is to use your eyes to be here, more available, and present—not to keep your eyes open all the time. You are welcome to shut them if you are feeling uneasy, tired, or when you simply need some alone time. If you do decide to close your eyes in this way, it is crucial to let your spouse know so that they are not left wondering where you went.

Keep in mind that using your eyes only serves to support you, not to cast you in a negative light. It's preferable to close your eyes and feel at ease with yourself if opening your eyes makes you feel so uncomfortable that your body feels far away. Try opening your eyes once more and notice how it feels when you are grounded in your body once more. If your eyes start to burn or start to tear up, there is likely a lot of strain there.

It will pass when your eyes start to relax from the sensation of being exposed, so don't panic. Constantly try new things to determine what works best for you. Hold your faces apart at a distance that both of you find to be comfortable. Some people find it challenging to focus up close. Speaking openly about what feels right and what doesn't can aid in relaxation, present-making, and awareness of the here and now.

Holding the space between you

I discovered that making love to my spouse face-to-face really helped me to be present. Because we are facing each other when we make eye contact, this may seem clear, but there is more to it than that. When I say "facing," I mean that you should keep your faces close together, about an inch apart, while being conscious of how near your partner's face is to yours. Do this when making direct eye contact is impossible and, more generally, when you need a break from it. The skin, chin, cheeks, brows, forehead, and profile can all be absorbed by the eyes as they retain the space between the faces. This infuses love with amazing sensuality. I saw, however, that I was noticeably less present when I pressed my face against my partner's neck, shoulder, or chest. It seemed comfortable and familiar, yet there was no struggle involved, making it simple for me to lose focus.

When I brought my head and spine back into alignment and put my face close to that of my partner, the sensation of restoring consciousness was wonderful as presence immediately filled the air. I discovered that I lost awareness of this moment whenever I crossed his midline, moved forward past his ear, turned my face away from his, or leaned to the side. It is possible to lose presence due to familiarity and associations with a certain method of embracing simply because we have grown accustomed to the embrace. By bridging the distance between you with your gaze, you can bring forth greater pleasure as consciousness permeates the body.

Let yourself enough time and space to explore with your eyes rather than setting restrictions and to accept your lover's sincerity and openness. Observe how receptive you can be and how much you can absorb of him through your eyes. See how far you can go by taking a close look at yourself. One day, a doorway will open and the sex center and eyes will come together. It's magnificent!

- Eyes are windows of the soul, a powerful channel for sex energy.

- Eye contact intensifies awareness of the present moment.

- "Soft vision" makes you receptive, open, brings intimacy.

- Close the eyes at times too; keep looking inward and downward.

CHAPTER SEVEN

THE BREATH

DO NOT FORGET TO BREATHE! Take slow, deep breaths. Breathing becomes utterly divine if you master it. It infuses the body with passion and sensitivity and catapults us into the experience of the present. Hence, the intentional use of the breath can significantly enhance foreplay and romantic relationships. Various therapies and approaches to breathing recommend certain and special breathing techniques, systems to follow, energy centers on which to focus, and where to breathe in and out, but I found it was best to keep it simple and remember to breathe.

I realized I was just paying attention to the in and out of everything until I tried to concentrate on a specific breathing pattern. My body's sensations, including the sense of taking in and absorbing the breath, were pushed to the side while my focus was focused on perfecting a breathing method. It is much better to simply be aware of the breath as it naturally goes in and out of you as a beginning point rather than trying to control it.

The breath can be seen as a link between the mind and the body, and becoming aware of its rhythm serves as a powerful anchor for the here and now. Switching from thinking to feeling is beneficial. If you have ever had the good fortune to focus just on your breathing, you may have realized that your mind was not present. You might even say that you went insane, lost all sense of reason, and were overcome by life's vitality and delight. This is so that breathing can reconnect us with our vital life force and free us from the mental aspects of sex or our thought processes. As we make love, we start to feel more tactile, sensitive, and sensuous. We can reach in between and around our cells and create a delicate porousness in the body by connecting with the breath and intentionally absorbing it.

Breathing and sexual vitality

When we are young, our normal breathing pattern massages the sex center. A wave is produced by a baby's effortless breathing and travels through to the lower abdomen and pelvic region. It pulses through the flexible diaphragm that divides the chest from the abdomen, pushing the organs below as a result, and then pulses into the pelvic floor. The genitals, which are made up of a complex network of muscles, act like a diaphragm that expands with each breath, continuously stroking the sexual organ. Our childhood breath becomes disturbed as we age due to tensions, repressions, guilt, and embarrassment related to sex, genitalia, or masturbation. The breath gradually stops passing via the diaphragm to the genitals or even the belly as the limit of the breath rises higher and higher.

The majority of adults are just using the upper portion of their lungs when they breathe, which limits the full benefits of breathing. This physical strain causes us to breathe shallowly instead of deeply, creating a barrier out of our fear of being open and vulnerable. When this happens, the genitals are devoid of the life force and food that comes from the breath that flows continuously downward into them.

This is why it's important to connect your breath, gut, and genitalia when you're in a romantic relationship. Receptivity and vulnerability are produced by relaxing the entire front and midline of the body, from the throat, heart, solar plexus, and low abdomen down to the genitals. You are aware of your surroundings right away, taking note of the elusive, pungent nighttime scents, unexpectedly happy bird songs, and the comforting moist chill of an early morning breeze.

It's amazing how disconnected from their breath most people are. Even though breathing is essential to life, we don't even realize we are doing it. My massage therapist kept telling me to breathe during our first session. It irritated me. As I finally lost patience, I yelled in rage how much I detested breathing. I wasn't a breath enthusiast when I first started learning about Tantra. But when I started to alter the way I made love and become more conscious of my breathing, I started to take deep, slow breaths.

After a few months, I began to detect a softening of the limitation and an upward push of the breath toward my belly and pelvis. It appeared to be forming its pathway to the genitalia. I found that I relished breathing more and more as I became more conscious of it. And the more I realized that breathing was a kind of internal massage that could improve my life, the more I wanted to do it!

Any attention you pay to your breathing before initiating a romantic relationship will make a significant effect. It might be as easy as focusing on your breath boundary while you get ready for a romantic evening in the shower. I observed that I rushed around until the very last minute when I was expecting my lover, making my home and I appear more hospitable. I was much better equipped to welcome him into a quiet space once I started to lie down and breathe deliberately five or ten minutes before he came. My body had been receptive due to breathing, and this femininity had established a striking appeal between us.

Breathing Into Love

It is advantageous to sit silently for a while before initiating a romantic relationship, much like in meditation, where the focus is inward. Ten to fifteen minutes will do.

You'll have a chance to tune into your body and become present during these periods of silence. Close your eyes and direct your focus downward as you sit, either by yourself or with your partner. Diaphragmatic breathing is how you should be breathing. The breath can also be thought of as traveling in a circle through the body, starting at the genitalia and moving up the spine, over the head, and down the front to the genitalia. Your inner environment is energized and sensitized when you concentrate on your breathing; this will trigger your sex energy when you begin to make love.

During sex, the breath's miraculous life-affirming phenomena drastically heighten presence, ecstasy, and pleasure. You should breathe in such that you can hear your breaths coming in and going out. This makes it easier for you to pay attention to your breath, and your partner can also hear it. In this sense, talking to one another and communicating through breath are both possible. Sometimes you and your spouse will unintentionally settle into a rhythmic breathing pattern where you both breathe in and out at the same moment. The feeling of breathing in the wonderful present moment will be wonderful.

We can refer to this coordinated breathing as "simultaneous breathing" if it is done voluntarily. Breathe in and out jointly while you pay attention to your partner's breathing pattern and learn to tune into it. Be at ease to foster rapport rather than stress, which will awaken the sex energy. It's crucial to never make breathing an effort, no matter what you try. You will go back to your thinking and miss the experience of your breath if you second-guess whether you should be taking an inhalation or an exhalation or if you are in harmony or not. Keep in mind that it is your awareness of the breath itself, not the act of taking a breath, that makes the difference.

Forming one breathing body

Another type of breathing, which we might refer to as "synchronous breathing," may also occur when two people are in a romantic relationship. The breath is circular in motion and has a significant impact on sex energy. When two persons are fully fused in sexual union, this breathing occurs rather naturally. As two become one breathing body in great empathy, it pierces right through your core. But, this type of deliberate breathing requires some mental work and can distract you from the present moment's urgency. But, give it a go for fun and see the results.

Continue to breathe slowly and deeply. If you'd like, after you've established the rhythm of this synchronized breathing, you can improve it by seeing the energies traveling in a circle.

The man exhales through his penis and inhales through his heart. She inhales through her genitalia and exhales through her heart. Consider the breath as a golden light that circulates in a circle. When the couple is sitting up together and the woman's legs are encircling her partner's pelvis, this can be quite attractive. The polarity within the bodies is enhanced by this close contact between the breasts and the chest.

Mouth breathing may assist you in becoming more fully aware of your body, even if breathing via the nose is more refined because it impacts the meditative and subtle body centers. Be free to use whatever method of breathing works best for you at the time because breathing via the mouth has an impact on the lower body centers and emotions. I would suggest inhaling through your lips if you are having difficulties "being here," distracted, or agitated about something else, as it might be helpful to eliminate the emotions that would otherwise impede awareness and presence. When you or your partner swallow frequently, it typically means that some sort of emotion is rising and the swallowing is an unconscious attempt to repress it. If you have a swallowing urge, attempt to relax into resisting it so that the suppressed energy can rise to the surface and exit. The effort required to overcome the reflexive want to swallow is significant, but it is well worth it. A stronger connection with your sexual energy is made when you allow the reflex action to be expressed, which may include tears, laughing, or even a violent cough.

Playing with your breathing

It is simplest to start with an out-breath as you start to focus on your breath. Forcefully expel all of the air from your chest. Once you've relaxed, the breath will forcefully enter your lungs and expand your chest in a wonderful in-breath. Hold your lungs empty for a few seconds. Breath becomes instantly conscious as a result. This instantaneous bodily awareness of the breath's vitality allows one to connect with the breath's flow both inner and outward. If you like, repeat this a few times while taking deep breaths that are slow and rhythmic.

Breathing in the other direction, deeply and slowly, will produce a comfortable environment for sexual energy because, typically, when we grow excited about sex and proceed toward climax and ejaculation, the breath will become shorter and faster. Tantra claims that there won't be ejaculation when lovers continue to breathe rhythmically and in harmony. The body never expels energy when the breath is rhythmic because it absorbs it.

You can occasionally inhale with a sniff, sniff, sniff motion. It's possible to take many quick sniffs before taking a full inhalation. Pause a moment and experience the breath's power to sustain life. then let out a breath. Short, sniffing breaths can be taken repeatedly to sharpen the awareness in the third eye and heighten the sensation of the breath entering the body. Play around and try some new things.

Consider the breath entering your body and enveloping each cell. Look into each other's eyes while you breathe to heighten the sensation. Make your breath-playing creative and exciting for yourself, whatever you choose to do it. So always keep in mind to feel your breath and continue inhaling into its confines. Imagine the blood absorbing the oxygen and providing more vitality as you breathe into the lungs and between the cells.

When you make love when in the most relaxed state, your consciousness merges with your breath, which becomes lighter, quieter, and sometimes even stops entirely. You take a breath, and it does not turn back. There is nothing wrong if this happens; it is a beautiful and silent moment. Breath is not required because there is no energy flowing outward at this time. Be suspended and allow yourself to simply be in this utopia, encircled by timelessness. The sexual energy will receive an unexpected push, rising upward and coursing ecstatically through the inner physical channels, and the respiration will naturally begin to pick back up. You and your partner will become one with life itself.

KEY POINTS:

- Breath has a profound influence on sexual energy.
- Breathe slowly and deeply while making love.
- Breathe downward through the diaphragm toward the genitals.
- Awareness of the breath creates the experience of the present moment.

CHAPTER EIGHT

COMMUNICATION

LOVERS COME TO SEE ME WITH TROUBLE OFTEN, NOT ALWAYS BECAUSE THE SESSION IS HARD, BUT BECAUSE COMMUNICATION IS A TRAP. They have a lot of disagreements and misunderstandings.

The priceless current moment is constantly disturbed by past events, conflicts, and concerns. They claim that they haven't made love for days or weeks because they have been preoccupied with blaming one another, attempting to establish who is right and who is wrong, and who is in control of whom, which has left them in a state of exhaustion and madness. Eventually, they are thankful for a break and fall asleep in each other's arms. When they awaken, they are ready to start over.

How To Express Your Feelings

The truth is that some people have a natural talent for expressing their emotions accurately. Others can't seem to convey their most enigmatic inner feelings and aren't even sure what they are feeling, much less when they are feeling it. Words may not form at all or may seem insufficient when emotions are intense. Regardless of communication skills, most individuals concur that sharing and being honest are delicate topics.

It can entail saying anything that appears to be against the person you love, or expressing that a specific touch did not feel good or wasn't appropriate at the time. How can we convey this information to our partner without offending them, coming out as judgmental, or as inflexible? We are all essentially insecure when it comes to sex, thus this might happen with ease. The ego's barriers can easily come between you, leading to discord and conflict rather than love.

Being sincere and telling the truth is crucial. You'll discover that the truth liberates your energy, causing you to become overflowing with vigor. Be mindful to choose your words carefully so that you may communicate with your spouse without offending them. Start by saying, "I feel," and then continue talking about yourself. Don't discuss them or what they did. If your body withdraws in response to your lover's touch, you are likely reacting to a combination of traumatic past sex experiences and not just to your current partner. In a tiny way, yes, but frequently the overload from the past is what's triggering the response. Very likely, this is not the first time it has occurred. Hence, you must be extremely aware of this when you speak to ensure that you are not taking revenge on everyone who has ever treated you unfairly (see chapters 22 and 23).

For instance, I frequently engaged in a particular foreplay approach that I knew would contract rather than increase my sexual energy to please a man, but it never worked. Every time I attempted to ignore my body's truth, I experienced malnutrition or lovelessness as a result. Maybe I made love with less awareness than I wanted to, leading to the same malnourished outcome. While it would be simple to point the finger at my partner for not meeting my needs or acting morally, the real culprit was my lack of honesty and integrity—specifically, my reluctance to be open and honest about what I liked. He wasn't to blame for my discontent; it was me!

While making love, communication is a powerful aspect. By bringing inner body sensations to the forefront, talking about what happens to you as you make love helps you ground yourself firmly in your body and this sexual experience. With the body, we are making contact with reality and so generating the present. Moving from the mind to the body, from thinking to feeling, and from doing to being is supported through communication.

We can turn our attention away from the racing mind and its thoughts and emotions by concentrating on the reality within the body, its various moods, and sensations. Communication is crucial because many of us are so preoccupied with our thoughts that we have little awareness of or control over our bodies. Tell your spouse what you are feeling in your body, where it is, and when it is happening. If you do this, you'll notice that you start to feel remarkably alive, perceptive, and present.

Sharing your present moment

Regrettably, conversations between people are rarely honest, especially when in a sexual position. If we did, a lot of issues would be resolved. Some couples do realize that they would never communicate this way, even in a romantic relationship. They start to realize that they constantly switch between planning, some distant memories, and hazy future wishes. I first had a lot of reluctance when I tried to talk in public about the present while in a romantic relationship, but I soon realized that the reason for my resistance was a fear of facing my own insecurities. I feared being exposed and his opinions of me.

Also, I was hesitant to explain how delighted I was about this opportunity, our exquisite body odors, the beauty that sparkled in his eyes, the supple, smooth, and silky skin, and the love that I could feel emanating from his penis. Like most things, it got easier the more I practiced. Speaking without inhibition was a comfort. My body got more lively as I freed up a lot of energy by telling my boyfriend the truth. I learned more about our genitalia, our physical characteristics, our sensitivities, our pleasures, and our insecurities. Communicating what is occurring as it occurs fosters closeness and unwavering openness, which makes it easier to be grounded in the body, attentive, and present with one another, which is where love flourishes.

I would advise you to express to your partner how you are feeling physically or emotionally and to be as explicit as you can. Never conceal anything. As you are having sex, keep up a calm conversation in which you both describe what is happening inside of you, pausing at leisurely intervals. The main notion is that by paying close attention to the present moment, we greatly increase our awareness of what is happening. And this alters the experience's overall quality. It gains consciousness and life thanks to it. To prevent yourself from daydreaming, avoid awkward or protracted silences. Employ language to draw both of you into the present moment. I refer to this as "sharing your present."

This creates a sincere foundation between you and grants newfound freedom. It is just a few words to honestly express the various feelings you are experiencing inside of your body, not a confession. Your consciousness and sensitivity will increase as a result, and your body's energy will also increase.

Feelings in your body

The fact that I could barely feel anything in my vagina when I stopped being so physically involved in lovemaking was one of the toughest things for me to confess. I was so accustomed to enjoying the sensations of friction that I was not yet capable of using the finer, more delicate ecstatic function or sensitivity. It was a horrifying moment when I had to admit to my lover that I couldn't even feel myself, let alone him! I felt like I was dead inside! After making this admission, I felt a great deal of sadness and pain overwhelm me.

I started crying and sobbing a lot, and as this energy was let go, I unpredictably felt more alive in my vagina. Unbeknownst to me, a layer of anxiety and stress had been building up in my vaginal tissue. I started giggling when I realized I was still alive. Never be too embarrassed to admit what is going on. If there is any lingering shame, let that be a sign to you that it is something you should talk about.

Two important things happen as you make love: you communicate and "share your now." In the beginning, you are creating the present via your bodies, a new foundation for the sexual experience, and getting to know each other's and your genitalia all over again. Also, and perhaps most importantly, you are opening a line of communication between your genitalia and your brain. Speaking aloud causes "what is" to become conscious, and it seems as though the area of the brain in charge of consciousness may actually "hear" what you are saying. The genitals will respond right away with thrilling sensitivity and increased consciousness by affirming the truth and accepting reality. You are laying the foundation for a new sexual intelligence in this way.

Talk about all of it

As you get more practice, you'll discover a technique to speak such that your partner is informed positively about how your body reacts and opens up. Although we are all alike, we are also unique. When you've warmed up, there may be things you like, but too much stimulation at first can typically result in a heated, orgasm-focused style of lovemaking. Alternately, the stimulation makes you less sensitive. As you get closer to one another, slow down. Spend some time sensing both your own and your partner's bodies. Find out what they enjoy and how they enjoy it. Moreover, plainly and kindly describe how and where someone touched you. Hold their hand in yours and demonstrate your preferred method to them. Speak about everything. When you are not making love, chat to each other about your experiences making love because this helps the consciousness immensely and is also the most interesting topic.

EXERCISE

Here is a little activity you may do with your partner to practice this style of communication for enhancing body awareness and the present moment:

Make eye contact while facing each other and lying comfortably apart. Spend some time tuning into your own body while also keeping an eye on your partner's body nearby. After a little while, start speaking while keeping as much of your body's sensations as possible. Talk about several bodily impressions or sensations that you can name. Let the woman first express what she physically feels. It could be a racing heart, a trembling in the stomach, or even a recurring worry or panic. The man can then describe what is occurring to his body, penis, and respiration. Talk just about what your body or heart is experiencing right now.

Ask fewer inquiries and avoid starting conversations. Seek your present moment by paying attention to your body, then describe it to your spouse. For a while, alternate speaking in this manner while sharing the present moment of your body. Keep it short and to the point; avoid awkward silences. Be mindful of your body's altering sensations. Avoid attempting to comprehend or evaluate with the mind. For instance, if your partner indicates they are afraid, avoid discussing the reasons behind their worry. By doing this, you take a step back from reality and the intensity of the present. Just keep expressing where and what you are experiencing to your partner. If something isn't happening, don't try to pretend it is by being explicit and real. Don't bring up things that have already passed or things that happened previously.

Please continue. Your body energy may start to become more dynamic over time, and you might start to experience a sense of physical attraction. If you maintain this informal conversational rapport, making love will come naturally.

Releasing fear and tension

The greatest time to express your sentiments and emotions is right as they are happening if you can do so. The potential and energetic intensity are gone if you wait. When you subsequently discuss it with someone, it will be like giving them a news report of what happened—just another narrative without the excitement of real life. Saying to your partner, "I'm frightened to relax, I'm terrified that nothing will happen," when you are feeling uneasy, for instance, will have a dramatic influence on you since it acknowledges your worry of nothing happening during sex. When you suddenly realize that you've been worried your breathing may become rapid, and you may experience tearing up, fear, or pain.

Unconsciously, there has been a great deal of strain within you. Yet, you were less "present" and ahead of yourself at the time, so you were unaware of it. The restrictive fear is now released from the energy system in a cellular manner and eliminated as a toxin, which is frequently reflected in the strong body odor given off during such occasions. Consciousness or presence is now introduced into the sexual act through communication and other means. Such a powerful encounter with reality alters reality and is eventually calming.

Love progressively replaces fears as they gradually go away. But if you talked about your fear later, it wouldn't change you in any positive way. I've lost plenty of chances to be open with the person I loved because I chose to hold onto my greatest fears. Yet I soon realized that I was depriving myself of greater happiness and life and that my fear of being exposed was a myth.

Opening up and taking chances only helped me get closer to my partner and myself.

My entire body and breath come alive when I am sincere and able to express what I am feeling. My body trembles, pulses, and vibrates in response to my courage and the truth. This helps me feel alive and know that I am just susceptible to myself and not to anyone else. I was the one who blossomed and shone after each time I got the courage to reveal my obscure concealed feelings rather than my boyfriend. He was undoubtedly moved, and it enabled him to become more open as well, but I stood to gain. Each exposure felt like the removal of a layer that covered who I was. I finally realized that my boyfriend is not to blame for my development, inner progress, or love. Instead, I am in charge of myself and everything depends on me.

It is not my lover's job that gives me life and sensitivity; it is my vulnerability and attitude. I discovered that I had to first become closer to myself to get closer to my beloved. We may determine how much love we are willing to accept into our life in this way. The greater the experience of Tantric connection, the more the personality's mask is tested and broken.

The sounds and silence of your body

You might experience periods when you are so engrossed in the stillness and brilliance of the present moment, the depth of your sensitivity, that it may seem nearly hard to drag yourself out of these delightful depths and speak. You don't have to force yourself to speak if this occurs to you. Continue to unwind in the calm and silence. We can use our voices in a variety of ways in addition to speaking. Sounds are wonderful in sex, and you can utilize them to express your enjoyment.

Avoid sounds that originate in the mind rather than the body by being aware of them. This frequently occurs during sex when we create sounds to amuse the other person or to appear to be enjoying ourselves. These sounds are not sexual. A mental sound is more likely to have a tinny, surface-level hollowness whereas a deeply sexual sound will have a resounding authenticity that engages you.

Allow the excitement and delight of your inner bodily sentiments to be expressed through sounds that come from your body. Try to connect the sound with the actual feeling you are experiencing and cause the sound to emanate from that. Because of how far down in your body your neck is, it feels as though the sensation is producing a sound that is vibrating and amplifying within you. Sex and sound are one.

KEY POINTS:

- Communication is crucial; be conscious of what you say, and how you say it.

- Share what you feel in body and heart as you experience it.

- Words bring immediate consciousness to bodies in the present.

- This gives new information about each other, body responses, a fresh foundation for love.

- To take a step closer to the other, you have to take a step closer to yourself first.

CHAPTER NINE

GENITAL CONSCIOUSNESS

CONSCIOUSNESS IN THE GENITALS is the ability to access your living self from the inside. During regular sex, we direct our attention outward toward the genitalia while making love, intensely holding it there to feel sexual pleasure. In reality, however, we frequently use the penis and vagina to achieve our desires while being unconscious of what is happening to us.

Tantra encourages us to relax into our genitalia rather than focus on them. Always keep in mind that the approach is relaxed and not stiff or forced. Instead, we focus on them and start to form an inner perception and sense of them. The sexual act becomes more conscious as a result of this inward focus, which also gradually raises awareness of the penis or vagina. It can be useful to visualize a fire or liquid warmth that fills the pelvic area, melting and softening the genitalia.

Our orientation is inward, and by holding the genitalia in awareness as we make love, and practice listening to them, we begin to see and experience them as the ones who create love rather than ourselves.

Slowing it all down nicely

Genital consciousness will automatically arise as a result of slowing down all sex-related actions since it allows you to feel the genital encounter. This may initially seem counterintuitive since you may be confused about how your penis or vagina can perceive anything without the friction we're used to. It may seem difficult or perplexing to stop moving or slow down. Yet, when you slow down, the sensitivity will rise, bringing more genital consciousness and an extraordinarily intense level of pleasure. There is too much activity when there is a lot of movement to sense the more delicate genital function.

By penetrating slowly and taking several long seconds to experience the vagina's yielding softness, opening, and giving way, you can create the environment in which you will make love together. Experience the entire beautiful phenomenon, including penetration and penetration. Nothing else compares to it! then slowly descend towards the inviting depths. It can take a while to complete this. When you reach the finish line, pause and wait. After some time, you might want to slowly exit the room and enter it again, or you might just want to sit still for a bit. Let yourself be fully enveloped by the vagina's sensation.

Think of your penis as a source of loving energy that you direct toward your spouse. Fluidity and sensitivity develop from this kind of calm, deliberate, and relaxed initial greeting by the genitalia, and the sexual act takes on an unforced feel. Without objectives, each sexual encounter becomes its world of love.

The vagina becomes less sensitive and the defense that is immediately erected within the vaginal walls increases the more a woman shifts her pelvis back and forth. It is at this point that a woman starts to disconnect her mind from her vagina as she moves faster and creates more friction as she approaches a climax, especially a clitoral orgasm. If she pays attention, she will see that as she thrusts and moves her pelvis to produce pleasure, the entire vaginal musculature is tight and tense. Simply put, the vagina becomes less sensitive and receptive as the environment becomes more constricted. The complementing female genitals are unable to fully receive energy from the penis at this time when the vagina's sensitivity should be at its peak.

Staying sensitive

Women can sink inward when they cease moving their pelvis, retraining the vaginal muscles and membranes to become softer and more sensitive. We can establish genital consciousness in this way. My girlfriend and I would initially test this out and ask, "How slow is slow?" I was re-orienting my vagina to feel the event of penetration, the opening, the surrender, and the receptivity as he moved one millimeter at a time as I relaxed. It was wonderful! He was becoming more adept at sensing the piercing, warm, welcome presence of God. That can initially feel like a Catch-22 for the man. He has always believed that his hard-earned habit of moving is what gives him and his partner sexual satisfaction. While some men find it simple to break this behavior, others find it difficult. That requires work. Yet it will be well worth it when a man can take a moment to slow down if he can just sit in the vagina and unwind into the space of no feeling. Sensitivity that has been lost will eventually return. He will ultimately begin to experience sensations other than friction, such as entering an electrical outlet or a highly magnetic environment. It's captivating!

Make love for yourself

Inverting your concentration is the key to establishing your consciousness in the genitalia. Put yourself first and foremost in your focus. This implies that during making love, you pull within yourself rather than projecting outwardly toward your partner. The energy goes down and back into the body's base as we impress it rather than express it. Consider your energy descending backward, moving vertebra by vertebra into the pelvis. Suddenly, we can visualize and experience the spine as an upward-flowing freeway that connects to the genitalia.

Most women will discover that they unintentionally hold their vaginas tight and flexed while making love when we bring consciousness to the vagina. Under the belief that doing so will increase the man's level of pleasure, many women deliberately purposefully compress and tighten the vagina. Women can now conduct vaginal workouts to improve their musculature's flexibility and strength. This stems from the widespread worry that the vagina would be overly lax or even large, possibly from stretching during childbirth, and hence less appealing. The utilization of friction to produce sexual pleasure has given rise to fallacies that are both fear and belief.

Yet, attentive and conscious genitals are crucial if couples decide to try Tantra. It will take some time for the vagina and penis to regain their deep-level sensitivity, but if the woman maintains a constant awareness of the vagina while remaining calm, receptivity is heightened and a stronger energy exchange takes place. True ecstasy in sex can only occur when the vagina receives the welcoming feeling that consciousness imparts to it. The sex act naturally lasts longer when performed in a calm and aware vaginal environment. The man must do the same thing by relaxing his anus and paying attention to his buttocks. He should also be aware of his tendency to tightly squeeze his anus.

Men who are insecure and fear losing or failing to keep an erection may experience tension in the anus. The worry will not go away by tightening the anus. As he presses his pelvic region and genitalia forward, it will distort his energy, constricting his genital consciousness and compressing his sexual experience. He will feel more rooted in the base of the penis by loosening the anus, which will also soften the entire pelvic floor and allow the sexual energy to "sink down and backward into the body." Men have described this sensation as making love from "behind" the penis, and many people have found this to be a very important Love Key since it helped to make the penis more sensitive and lengthen the intercourse.

Be aware of your pelvic floor

The majority of people have no idea what the pelvic floor is, where it is, or what it does. One of the males in the course of my couple said that he had no idea he had a pelvic floor until three days prior. He was now unable to ignore how tense the situation was. In actuality, we hardly ever feel down into the tissue of our genitals. The only time we allow ourselves to feel "down there" is when we are having sex or masturbating, and even then, just a little. Unbeknownst to us, we have a long-standing tendency of keeping our distance from the genitalia. We grip our sex centers tightly in an unconscious manner all the time. As stated in chapter 2 on sexual conditioning, we are tightening the pelvic floor muscles, which hold the genitals in constant corkscrew tension. Moreover, this strain prevents the breath from pumping into the pelvic floor.

The lovely base of the torso is made up of a web of muscles that extends across the base of the pelvis and connects to the sit (buttock) bones, pubic bone, and coccyx. The genital organs are formed from and enmeshed in these intertwining muscles. Some muscles can be utilized to intentionally contract the anus, and there is another set of muscles that can stop urine flow, tighten the vagina, or flick the penis. The perineum, located behind the vagina or the root of the penis in front of the anus, is another key area of the pelvic floor. When you tighten up, the musculature pulls up like a parachute into a central, tangled tendon that you can feel with your hand. You will feel a bump under your touch. Particularly here, our stresses build up, trickle down, and have an impact on the energy and structure of the legs and feet. The abdominal floor is being continuously raised by us. Every time you focus on your pelvic floor, you'll find that you may relax it and release it, which may cause the musculature to recede two to three cm! The primary feature of the pelvic floor is that it is constantly being pulled up, tightened, and constricted. Furthermore, we are completely unaware of this central tension. It has been a constant reference point since I learned about my pelvic floor, which was at least fifteen years ago. I began bringing my attention to my pelvic floor, and I would discover that I was holding it tense each time. As I would intentionally let go of it, my body would exhale in relief and I would feel more at peace since my legs and feet would be in closer contact with the ground. I would return there moments or minutes later to discover that it was crowded.

No matter how many times I intentionally let go, the instant I lost awareness, my unconsciousness, my anxiety, and the tension I carried around sex would draw upward to tighten. I asked a close friend of mine if she ever felt any tension in her pelvic floor because I remember it particularly irritating me at one point. She replied, "Never!" I was shocked to learn this! Was I truly so anxious? greater than most? We reconnected a while later, and nearly the first thing she said was: "When I last saw you, I haven't stopped feeling my pelvic floor! I was unaware that I had never been aware of it."

Expand the muscles of your pelvic floor

As you are making love, gently relax your pelvic floor to improve your genital awareness. First of all, identify it while standing. Tighten up all the muscles surrounding your genitals and anus, pretending you are preventing the flow of pee. It's easy. Squeeze a bit tighter, to accentuate the tension. Tighten the muscles and then let it go, relax. Visualize that you are bottoming out, emptying via the vagina or penis and anus. Let the energy run down the legs. Experience the new inner feelings that come with this. Try this out and then do it as frequently as possible.

Do it anywhere, while in a line, while speaking at a cocktail party, it's okay—nobody can see you, and it feels amazing! Suddenly you will find yourself more at ease, more confident with a feeling of belonging. Make this an awareness practice that you perform again and again since it promotes vigor to the pelvic region. But do not do it mechanically or subconsciously, else it makes the vagina harsher. Feel instead that you are maintaining it in tone, balance the pushing up with the letdown, do it carefully millimeter by millimeter, and notice how the awareness expands. The beauty of consciousness is that it knows no limitations. Women may always discover another layer of awareness in the vagina by pressing the mind into the vagina and asking themselves, "Can I be more open?" Amazingly the musculature will expand a few millimeters, and as the very cells are penetrated with awareness, the male penis will react with jerking spasms, slithering deeper deeply into the vagina.

Males may hold the full penis in awareness, not merely the very magnetic sensitive tip. Experience its whole length as it expands magnificently out from the body. Additionally feel the root of the penis where your penis attaches and exits from the body, and the perineum, the little knotty region between the penis and the rectum. This is the epicenter of the male positive pole, thus a guy should continuously maintain the root of the penis at the forefront of his mind. Don't concentrate on where it is (it might stimulate excitement), but on how it feels; this develops the internal awareness of the penis. Remain connected with this and feel or imagine the penis to be a rod or a magic wand. The higher the awareness present in the penis, the more you will be able to depend on its intellect. The penis will instruct you how to make love, when to stay motionless, when to move, and how much to move, in direct relation to the environment inside the vagina.

The fact is that most men seldom experience the complete length of the penis since the attention is on the feeling being generated in the tip, generally by repeated quick motions. Yet when they do, they have found it to provide an instantaneously enlarged character to the sexual energy, the sense of oneself via the penis with strength coming from the root, conveyed along the base upward and enhancing the sensitivity of the head, its magnetic qualities. This is helpful for both men and women since the more sensitive the penis head, the more delicate and blissful vibrations inside the vagina may be sensed. This finer magnetic genital functioning is the gift of Tantra, a very rewarding and therapeutic experience for men and women.

KEY POINTS:

- Inner focus, slower movements, feeling the genitals from within brings consciousness to them.
- Relaxing the pelvic floor repeatedly allows the sexual energy to configure and expand.

CHAPTER TEN

TOUCH

IMAGINE THE BODY AS A HUGE delicious fruit with soft and luscious sections all over it. You know them, you have felt them in your own body.

So how can you touch and remain aware such that it delivers maximum pleasure to you and your lover? Stroking and stroking your sweetheart as much as possible provides you the opportunity to experience the sexual effects of touch. Observe the small reactions to your touch and be directed by it. Touch gently with awareness in your hands. While you are being caressed, shut your eyes and allow yourself to feel the contact. Absorb the warmth into your own body.

Touch and be touched when you make love, it helps greatly to heighten sensuality and generate sexual presence.

I have discovered that any form of massage between lovers is a fantastic approach to beginning to make love. When massage is done with love and understanding, it swiftly generates relaxation, the lowering of tensions, and induces intimacy and rapport. Massaging the legs and buttocks has the effect of arousing sexual energy, particularly in women, who tend to keep unexpressed sexual energy in the upper legs, thighs, and buttocks. Sometimes this unexpressed sexual energy is mirrored in the bodily structure, resulting in excessive heaviness in the thighs. When awareness is introduced to lovemaking, being touched inwardly and outwardly, the body may experience enormous transformations, replacing imbalance and congestion with balance and fluidity. When the sex energy flows upward to the heart, gently we become merged into one elegant whole.

The dilemma is, how to touch it and where? The body is plenty of scrumptious touchable regions and wherever is an excellent location to touch, providing your partner agrees. We all know our bodies and the position of the most sexually sensitive spots, but I propose that you do not confine your caresses to such locations; it is best to approach them indirectly. Start with a peripheral body part, possibly the feet, the arms and hands, and the head, gently circling inside and lightly into the back, buttocks, belly, and more sensitive parts. This fosters trust and closeness and the slowness of the approach produces a sensuality and new awareness inside the bodies. You will observe your lover's body react favorably in gratitude. Fire develops slowly but definitely, and it requires nurturing. It is very possible that your body will be reacting in the same manner too. By contact there develops a physiological longing to make love together, and this alters everything.

Frequently when we touch one another, we will repeat the same action or caress again and again. Rubbing up and down, or round and round effortlessly, almost forgetting that we are in fact, touching the flesh. This lack of mindfulness in the touch might regrettably have an annoying impact on the recipient. She immediately senses the absence of awareness in the hand where there is no tactile contact and thus, without sincerity and sensitivity, there is no joy in it. Although your objective may be to turn your partner on, she may be turning it off instead. We may all prevent this by keeping attentive and mindful when touching.

Communicating through touch

Feel the exquisite curves of the body, the soft skin, the silky hair, the bony protrusions. As you are touching, don't concentrate so much on the doing, such as stroking or rubbing, but rather on the sensation of the contact between your hand and their body. Let your awareness penetrate your hand. Relax into being and envision your hand melting or dissolving into their body. The attention on the touch of the hand itself, rather than the action or the doing, affects the overall character of the contact. That is amazing. It allows your partner time to feel you, and integrate your touch into their body. You will discover that your companion heats up and reacts much more rapidly if your touch is mindful.

Feel yourself feeling them, and they feel it too. The sacrum, for example, is usually an excellent spot to touch. It feels wonderful! With a warm open palm convey your love into the base of the spine. It is a holy area. Feather-light strokes up the spine increase bodily energy considerably. Wrapping the entire, open hand around the back of the neck softly is highly soothing and reassuring, and this delicate touch may also aid in the discharge of tears. Or try putting both hands precisely on each of the sitz bones, the buttock bones on which we sit. Cup them completely, and to the one receiving, this warmth seems incredibly sensual. Take time to seek and uncover particular locations, and juicy spots, and learn how your beloved reacts. Use your hands to convey and show your affection.

While you touch your partner with mindfulness, imagine that you are flowing love and warmth into their body. This imagination enables you to obtain the impression of energy going from you into them and promotes communication. Hold your hands in one spot for a while, be glad to appreciate the simple touch. Don't do, "be." This form of attentive contact, without the purpose to arouse or thrill your partner, encourages them to direct their concentration inside to feel themselves. It promotes receptivity and sensitivity.

For instance, males may be guaranteed that devoting fifteen or twenty minutes to tenderly touching their partner's breasts or legs before entering her offers significant returns. It will bring you both to higher heights of pleasure and bliss. In serving a woman, a guy is satisfied as a man.

Touching the heart through the breasts

Considering our background Love Key, Polarity, it is vitally necessary that the breasts of a woman be caressed before and during lovemaking. Her positive pole has to be aroused before the negative pole, the vagina, reacts with sexual enthusiasm. When the female focus is on the clitoris or vagina, and the breasts are ignored, the sexual experience is more likely to be limited to a more linear genital one. When the positive pole, the breasts and heart of woman, is actively engaged, the sexual act takes on a different characteristic. It becomes round and spontaneous as a deep flow of sexual energy becomes attainable.

During making love, most women wish to have their breasts stroked with love and compassion. They intuitively know that it is the breasts that access the deeper layers of sexual energy. As I began becoming more cognizant of the function of the breasts during sex, I realized that much to my surprise, they were not particularly responsive. My connection with them had always been from the outside, and how they appeared as objects, rather than from any interior awareness or knowledge of them as breasts. This rendered them hypersensitive and unable to absorb the warmth of loving touch. I noticed that if the breasts and particularly the nipples were handled too violently or aggressively, it would have the effect of turning me off and causing my body to retreat, making me less inclined to make love. On the other hand, when they were caressed in a purposeful or more aware manner without the goal to excite, the contact would send sparks into my vagina. I opened up there and then! Later, when everything was rolling, there would frequently come a point when my breasts would be begging for a greater grip or contact and that would continue to expand my sexual energy.

I have talked to many women who previously enjoyed having their breasts stimulated when young, then reached a point where they no longer liked to have them touched. They were bloated, congested, or over-sensitive, and the nipples exceedingly reactive. What might happen is that the breasts, and hence the lady as well, become repulsed by insensitive contact done without empathy. Often, when a guy touches a woman's breasts, he is acting from his desire and excitement and not responding to the breasts themselves. He is caressing them in a manner that is nice for him, but not for her sexual reaction. A forceful touch could be more acceptable at some point later during lovemaking, but at the beginning, be deliberate and gentle. Intend to touch your spouse, and then contact with purpose. That makes all the difference.

Let your desire, admiration, love for your partner's breasts be conveyed via your hands. Breasts, the emblem of fertility, are undoubtedly gorgeous and have caught the eyes and emotions of the artist and the lover for all of mankind. Take the full breast into the palm of your hand, conveying energy and love. Don't do anything for a time, merely "be" with the breast in your palm, possibly delivering a slight squeeze now and again. Afterward stroke or lick the nipples lightly, in a childish fashion.

Listen to the energy of the breasts and feel how they would want to be caressed, not how you would like to touch them.

Free your normal method of responding to the breasts and nipples, and even your conditioned reaction to breasts. Caress them with the concept of reaching inside your lover, opening her heart in preparation for love. Enter the moment via the presence of your hand.

Caressing the penis

Similar to how a man should hold his penis in his hand, a woman should do the same. She should embrace her penis with her hand like she would a young, hardy bird. Once more, it has nothing to do with anything. Simply be there with it, taking in all of its wonderful energy, power, and softness. Take the testicles into your hands and carefully caress them, treating them like the most precious of eggs. Slowly draw the testicles out from the body while massaging them between the thumb and forefinger. The length of the shaft of the penis can be seen by slowly pulling back and away from the head of the penis the foreskin and other folds of skin.

It feels wonderful and aids in bringing the man's consciousness to his penis. The male can direct his attention, in particular, to the positive pole at the base of his penis. It will result in a vivid relaxation in a man's body when you use your hands to interact with his root. A stimulating touch, on the other hand, will emphasize the excitement component of sex, which encourages "doing" or climax.

Energizing the positive poles of love

Be in your hands and channel energy via them when you touch any part of your body. Anytime it feels like the proper time, give someone a tender, loving squeeze. Mutual touching of the positive poles can be utilized to start making love and has excellent success. Your sweetheart will be able to concentrate on his or her breasts or penis thanks to your exquisite touch, which awakens the sexual energy without stimulation. You can accomplish this by kneeling next to the woman who is lying down or by lying on your sides with your backs to each other. Put your relaxed hands on your partner's positive pole as you reach out to them.

Allow the eyes to contact and send your warmth and love to them through your hands. Before you start making love, stay in this mutual exchange for ten to fifteen minutes. Finding a position where you can be both comfortable and able to touch each other at the same time can be challenging. If so, touch each other while the other receives. then trade. make love after that.

Recall that this emphasis on the polarities of love that are good is crucial because it prepares the ground for the interaction of polarities once penetration takes place. An amazing energy exchange is conceivable when the opposing poles—the penis and vagina—are attuned to one another. Love can grow more and more energetic, with the bodies moving about and into each other for hours on end as if they were possessed by life itself.

Keep in mind that telling your partner how you are feeling physically when they are touching you can be very useful. Have a conscious dialogue with your body using a few short sentences to heighten your awareness.

Share yours now!

Don't think of contact as being limited to the hands alone. Be conscious of how and where the bodies actually touch, as well as the silky, slippery sensations between the legs, arms, lips, bellies, and chests. Be careful not to force your bodies too tightly against each other during the initial embrace and kiss. Unfortunately, this has the undesirable effect of compressing the physical body and the energy field that surrounds it, which restricts or eliminates any sensual emotions. Because the body won't permeable enough, consciousness won't be able to pass through it. They'll be regarded as substantial, immovable objects, which restricts receptivity.

Very certainly, when you embrace someone, you have experienced this difference. Without any genuine warmth or energy exchange, one person may give you a hug, a handshake, or even a slap on the back that leaves you gasping for air. You might be surprised when someone just melts into your arms. You feel vaporous and light all of a sudden, expanded by the contact. Out of the plainness comes a lovely tenderness.

According to Tantra, touch starts with you and takes a patient, sensitive approach so that the body's cells might blossom with energy and life. As you lie down, give yourself some time to feel yourself. Take a few deep breaths, then face your partner. Recognize the area that unites and divides you.

Let the eyes touch, then slowly bring the bodies closer together. It takes time and peace for more subtle phenomena to develop, which helps the body's environment support energy and electricity. The relaxed sexual energy can develop into a spontaneous and dynamic power when your bodies are touched in a sensitive, permeable, and mindful way.

KEY POINTS:

- Touching, stroking and caressing is a natural expression of love.

- Use relaxed friendly hands, conscious and slow, molding to the body curves and shapes.

- Channel energy and warmth through the hands to access the female sexual energy through the breasts.

- Receive the warmth radiating from a loving hand, accept and absorb the touch into your body.

CHAPTER ELEVEN

RELAXATION

ACTIVITY, EFFORT, and stress help us accomplish our goals, carry out our plans, and complete our projects. We develop a more loving heart and a stronger sense of well-being through relaxing. Most of us yearn for relaxed conditions where we have profound inner peace, each moment is joyful, and there are no bothersome or worrying thoughts about the future. To facilitate a more nutritious and loving exchange during sex, we are learning to relax in a variety of ways as we explore the Love Keys. We discover that we may start to relax once we let go of the notion that we must gain something from sex. Orgasms are no longer the ultimate prize that must be obtained by constant effort and strain. It's good when it happens, yet it's also good when it doesn't.

When there is no pressure to make things the way they should be, acceptance of what arises. This acceptance results in realizing and appreciating what is happening, including the lovely pleasures of the body, the straightforward breath, the feelings that come and go, and the alertness that arises with an inward focus. All of this leads to profound sexual relaxation. When we are in this mindset, we are ready to accept whatever happens next, nearly purring like a cat and entirely attentive to our changing environment.

All of us have admired cats' excellent awareness while envious of their serenity. To transform the sexual act from a rigid routine into a mystical unfolding, we must add relaxation. We must revert to our childhood selves, completely engrossed in the seashells that line the sparkling coastline. Many of us, whether consciously or unconsciously, find ourselves looking for ways to recapture this lost serenity and engrossment from infancy at some point in our lives.

The power of doing less and being more

It's common to describe the exhausted or lazy condition in which you're uninterested, bored, disengaged, or drowsy and sleepy as one of relaxation, but it's not. With relaxation, you come back to Earth renewed rather than destroyed. The process of relaxing involves waking up more and more. It is an effective force. If you've ever had the endearing sensation of a tiny newborn encircling your finger with a firm grip of life energy, you've experienced the power of a child's lack of muscular strength to relax. When you shift your focus from the outside to the inside, from the external to the internal, from activity to rest, and from doing more to being less, you can truly relax. You will realize how revitalizing it is if, when you lie down to rest in the afternoon, you slowly and deliberately relax different portions of your body and then stay in that awareness for fifteen or twenty minutes.

Releasing tension renews the body and energizes the spirit. You change when you come out. Crucially, unlike what many people believe, relaxing involves returning presence to the physical structure rather than the collapse of the physical structure. Consciously relaxing makes you enter your body, which then makes you more awake, energetic, sensitive, and receptive. That is more of a checking in than a checking out. Therefore, when you make love, you don't just vanish and leave your partner; rather, you show up in your body, poised and ready.

The body exhibits tension, which is the opposite of relaxation, as hardness in the muscles and other body tissues. Having worked on innumerable bodies in therapeutic massage clinics over the years, I've discovered that the majority of people's upper backs, shoulders, and necks feel like solid, dense concrete, giving them a sense of extreme density. Because of internal and external pressures, the body's cells are compressed, leaving insufficient room for physical comfort.

Too many people describe being exhausted and anxious, as well as having neck pain, headaches, eyestrain, and breathing and sleeping issues. Physical discomfort has a significant impact on our psychological state and can quickly determine whether we are happy or unhappy. Physical therapies are a solution since they promote both physical and mental relaxation, but an hour of exercise or a massage won't undo years' worth of built strain. The process of relaxing keeps getting deeper and actually never ends. The majority of our bodies have lost this soft, watery aspect. The body is made up of 70 to 80 percent water, making it seem like a giant elastic bag and somewhat jelly-like. The body can return to its fluid, supple state through awareness and relaxation.

Convincing ourselves that relaxation has real value may be the hardest part of the process. Is doing so advantageous? How many times have you considered taking a nap but your mind quickly told you that you needed to be doing something else? So you completed a chore that had been waiting for you for a long time, something you could later celebrate. Even so, you might have felt terrible for spending the morning in bed, thinking it was time squandered or poorly spent. In our life, there is no intrinsic value placed on relaxation. Even more strongly, sex exhibits the same kind of urge to act.

Giving up control for expansion

Hence, with our new method of lovemaking, we have to bring relaxation by minimizing the amount of physical effort we exert. It entails relaxing the body and its actions (slowing down to reach genital awareness), and it also implies relaxing the mind. At this time it is frequently hard to imagine that forgetting about orgasm and opting to rest instead is going to be rewarding! Our thoughts, our sexual programming, our prior experiences, will frantically persuade us out of relaxing, by saying "Go for it, it's so great anyhow, what could be better?" In fact, by relaxing, we are abandoning our power over the sexual act, and the components of our sexual expression that keeps us tied into routines.

It is not so simple for the mind to accept the thought of less control, therefore reason will be determined to keep you confined and inside your regular spectrum of experience. But, when we finally manage to relax below the drive for a climax or "doing," we will find the experience full of richness and diversity. It astounds me how many levels of relaxation are available. Just when I think my body or mind is entirely relaxed, I detect still an extra layer of subtle tightness. With each descent into relaxation, there is a matching sensation of expansion inside the body, awareness of increasingly delicate vibrations. There develops a sensation of bright and porous vitality at an intercellular level.

While you make love, wander over your body again and again to identify any regions of tension, the locations where you are involuntarily clenching your muscles. It might be the shoulders, the inner thighs, the feet, the tummy, the mouth, or the anus.

Anywhere. Each drop in relaxation counts. Tightness in the jaw is generally associated with tension in the pelvic region, so again and again bring your focus to the jaw and relax it when you make love. That is well worth it. When you play about relaxing various regions of the body in this manner, you will discover how the slightest of tensions effect your sexual energy. When you release them, even if there seems to be no direct association between the bodily parts, for instance, the shoulders and the penis or the feet and the vagina, you will sense an increase in sexual feelings.

But unlike the pelvic floor, the solar plexus too is a region to relax and imbue with awareness, particularly while you make love. Here too, we accumulate and store various unconscious tensions including the crippling impacts of traumatic emotional events. That is consequently not an area in which we have much awareness.

Nevertheless, when the solar plexus is relaxed and filled with awareness, the sexual interchange between man and woman transforms. It brings actual spontaneity into the sex act and helps you to keep the awareness inside while being totally attentive to the outside happenings. This region may not be easy to perceive at first, or it may produce sensations of nausea or a lump in the stomach, a definite indicator of concerns and tensions stored in the body. With time these bad sentiments are released. Once it is easier to reach this place, it is a recommendation to lovers that they retain their consciousness in the solar plexus when they make love.

The fire of awareness created up here flows warmth over into the genitals. When we are present, we are actually impassioned. This contact with the solar plexus has the power to press away the tired ideas through which we constantly filter our experience. There is a powerful impression of being inside and outside simultaneously. Guys pleasantly say that the impulse to ejaculate reduces, and there is an ease and relaxation from which power develops.

Relaxing into sexual energy

The reaction to relaxation is natural; we are born with it. I sometimes call it the sixth sense. If one person is entirely calm and present the other person will instantly be impacted and become more relaxed and present themselves. For instance, when a woman relaxes profoundly in lovemaking, without really doing anything but focusing on receiving and being present instead, naturally her spouse will become more aware, sensitive, and loving. He will instinctively connect with the moment, and thoughts of orgasm will not even surface.

Instead, a magical portal opens and the guy experiences something altogether different occurring to him. That is an unforgettable experience. For the first time he has been able to make love without effort or strain. It is more of a dance, a sensual interweaving of bodies. Therefore never feel that you must wait for the other to relax before you can; relaxing begins with you first and foremost.

Accumulated tensions kept in the body have a tiring impact on it, so when couples modify the way they make love and begin to relax, they frequently describe feeling extremely exhausted, true drowsiness, the urge to collapse or an actual physical weakening in the muscles. Maybe they even feel low blood pressure. This is a solid indicator that relaxation is begun. The old tensions are rising through exhaustion, and that is not a reason for fear. The persistent unfelt exhaustion emerges sharply, and in this manner is removed from the body. That is extremely useful. Take lots of rest, and do not be in a rush to get someplace or do anything. When relaxation in sex is accomplished, it is the closest you can deliberately go to the base of your energy system. Relaxing here at the root will have a ripple effect on every level: mind, body, and soul. The advantages are virtually instantaneous without needing to do more or less than make love.

In essence, when we are no longer hooked or driven by our sexual cravings, when mind and body can completely relax into the present moment and its splendor, we feel the backflow of our sexual energy. Instead of straining it to a release, we relax and allow the energy to languidly fall back on itself, and then ascend within and upward. In this approach relaxing is fundamental to Tantra. It demands a slow and timeless approach; if you have made love for three or four hours or more, you will feel the profound sense of calm and love it provides. This special trait emanates from inside you.

An effortless surrender

Time is only essential when we have an aim to complete, someplace to go. Without such ambitions, there is simply no reason to rush. You may relax and take a long, languid stroll, relishing sensuous sensations and thus boosting sex to a new frequency.

By this relaxation, the sexual energy is reabsorbed by the body. Set aside a few hours so that you do not have to worry about the time since time usually causes strain. With this, relaxing will be easy. Be playful, touch, caress, kiss. Take time to know each other physically and allow an attunement to grow between the bodies, let it be a slow, gradual coming together. What we are aiming to build inside our bodies is a serene atmosphere, not an exciting one. It's a vital step if you intend to explore with sex as an uplifting force. That is the difference between pleasure and ecstasy! In making the first effort of not attempting sex, a sort of ease comes, surrendering to the life force as it starts to travel through the bodies with magnetic intelligence, seeking and searching completeness via the other. When we relax more and more into sex, we discover the refreshing characteristic of relaxation saturating our life, making us attentive, joyous, loving, and creative.

KEY POINTS:

- ❧ Sexual energy functions best in a relaxed environment.
- ❧ Use awareness to search for, and relax, unconscious tensions.
- ❧ Reduce the amount of physical effort in sex.
- ❧ The more you relax, the more the other person relaxes, deepening the experience.

CHAPTER TWELVE
SOFT PENETRATION

SINCE THE SEXUAL ORGANS are full of the accumulated stress of previous experiences, they are no longer able to operate according to their real polarity. Having lost their original sensitivity, the vaginal walls are not discovered to be in their normal condition; wet and slippery like the interior of the oyster. Instead of the softness one experiences while eating soft squishy coconut, they have grown stiffened and unyielding from years of friction. In the same manner, a man's penis, which in its normal form is snake-like, strong, and flexible, may become stiff and unyielding, almost metallic, as it expands, full of energy that cannot be appropriately funneled into a woman.

This tension in the genitals, which has impacted the male and female polarity, must gradually be released and cleared out so that the natural polarities may be restored. The penis must once again become a vehicle for creating and transferring energy to a woman, while the vagina becomes capable of welcoming, absorbing, receiving, and circulating this masculine energy. As the penis and vagina become more relaxed, free of their restricting tensions, the positive energy of the male and the negative energy of the female begin to challenge each other, with a pushing and pulling effect, creating a delicate and ecstatic magnetic sexual exchange, far more penetrating than the pleasures of friction-based sex could ever be.

A smart method to start restoring polarity is to try mild penetration—yes, without an erection! This thought is typically received with ridicule and incredulity, but it is a truth, the penis can go inside when it is not erect and it feels incredibly great. It may be inserted by the lady or the male. Furthermore, gentle penetration also removes the strain off the male by disproving the belief that the penis must be erect to make love. Getting to put the relaxed penis in the vagina is a talent that takes some experience, but it is well worth it. Additionally, if a guy is experiencing trouble getting an erection without stimulation, or if he suffers from impotence, gentle penetration implies that he may still enter a woman and make love to her.

When the penis is placed in its relaxed condition, the guy is given the chance to be more present, as the pressure of needing to have an erection may frequently lead to psychological anguish or sexual fantasy. With mild penetration, this pitfall is avoided. In traditional sex, the guy, according to his positive polarity, will normally be ready for sex far before the woman whose sexual temperature is naturally lower. By delicate penetration, this disparity may be bridged, and the man and woman can warm up together, the genitals softly welcoming and expanding into fullness.

The penis may get erect within the vagina in direct reaction to the vaginal environment, which provides a different type of sexual energy than that of penetration with erection. The genitals have an opportunity to attune to each other without the strain of needing to make anything happen. This absence of pressure to perform starts to restore equilibrium to the penis and vagina; stored tensions are flushed out, progressively returning to their naturally receptive condition.

Take the time to love consciously

It is likely that in the beginning, it may be impossible to feel anything at all in the penis or the vagina, much alone anything fascinating or delightful. Now you are in a gap. Imagine that someone is caressing your back furiously for many minutes and then abruptly stop. It wouldn't be that simple to sense the still hand at first. It would take a long to notice the energy and warmth traveling from the hand into your back since it is incomparably more subtle than the heat caused by the friction of rubbing. Likewise, if the genitals are used to friction as a manner of communicating, the contrast of no movement or decreased movement will initially provide less emotion.

The mild tingling electrical sensitivity between the penis and vagina during gentle insertion is so sensitive, it takes some time to get into the sensation of it. It is surely worth every second of waiting, however, since after a while the genitals begin to buzz together, and the image of sex as some type of action or an effort starts to shift.

A guy committed to conscious love remarked, "Before I experienced simple gentle penetration, the penis did not have any genuine feeling of a significant direction." He observed that when he relaxed deliberately while being soft within the vagina, his penis would gradually get erect as if dragged up into the depths of the vagina with an intelligence of its own. This innate orientation of the penis is an electromagnetic phenomenon and it is not anything you can "do." In reality, it is our "doing" that stops it from occurring. If a couple can relax with mild penetration (see fig. 7), and improve their genital awareness and presence, they will start to find a new level of sexual pleasure with the penis acquiring snake-like properties as it writhes ecstatically into the vagina, sucked inward by the opposite polarity. The more mindful you are while you make love, the more effortlessly the innate polarities will be restored to the genitals.

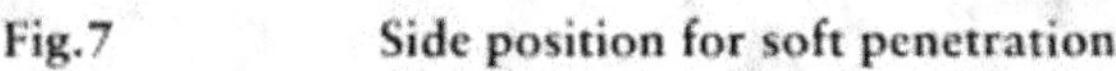

Fig.7   Side position for soft penetration

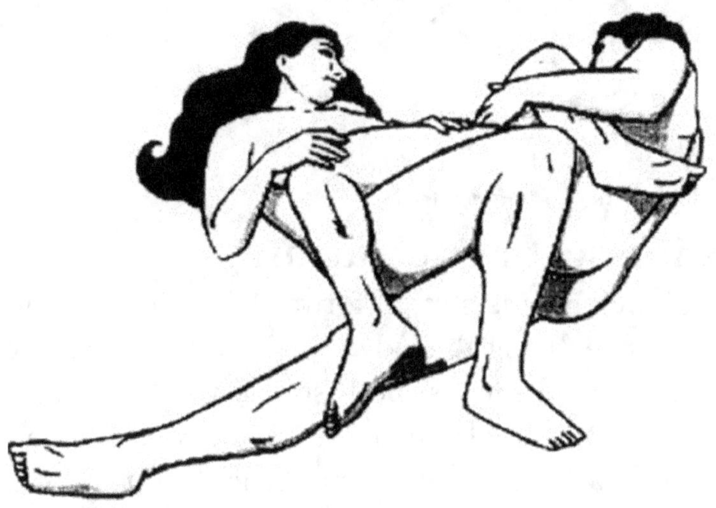

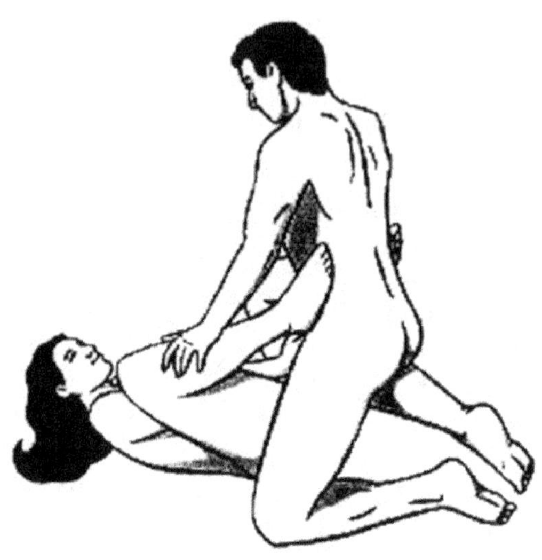

Fig.8   Middle position for soft penetration

Positions for soft penetration

The place for gentle entry is straightforward (see fig. 7). The male rests on his side facing the lady. The lady sleeps on her back, placing her pelvis near his. Both spread their legs, and the genitals will be naturally laying opposite one other. Bring them together, then wrap your legs around each other. This is sometimes dubbed the scissors pose. The woman may have to shift her upper body away from her lover's to make the pelvises meet, or she may slant her pelvis upward. Explore and do what is most comfortable. This may not work for every relationship. Laying between the legs of the lady for gentle penetration, and rolling onto the sides from time to time, is a nice option. At this medium position (see fig. 8) it is easier for a guy to enter the penis.

How the woman inserts the penis

For soft penetration in the side position, after you are positioned appropriately, with pelvises close together, with the vagina opposite penis, the woman may continue with the soft penetration by grasping the penis in her hands (see fig. 9). If you need lubrication, this would be the right opportunity to apply it but don't make it too slick to handle. Gently draw back the folds of the foreskin around the head of the penis, and expose it with the skin pushed away and down toward the root. Now construct a two-pronged fork with the first two fingers of each hand (short fingernails ideally!) Put one finger fork (try the left hand) firmly around the base of the penis and keep it there. With the other hand (the right) insert the fingers immediately on each side and beneath the rim enclosing the head of the penis. Pinch the fingers together so that you have a delicate grasp on the penis, and then bring the penis toward your vagina. As it reaches the entrance proceed to insert it. You will be able to push it in and up a little way. Do the same thing again.

Hold the penis between your two fingers, and guide it into your vagina. By repeating the finger action again and again, it is as if you're feeding or strolling the penis into the vagina, softly pushing it within a little further each time. After you have put all of it within you (or as much as you can manage to insert—even to get the head in is a good start), withdraw your hands, and pull the pelvic regions together as nearly as possible, then wrap your legs around each other and relax! Utilize cushions to make yourself as comfortable as you can, and use additional Love Keys to support your presentation. In this posture, eye contact is simple and crucial, as is breathing, and it is feasible also for the guy to lay a hand on the woman's breasts while she may touch his buttocks and thighs.

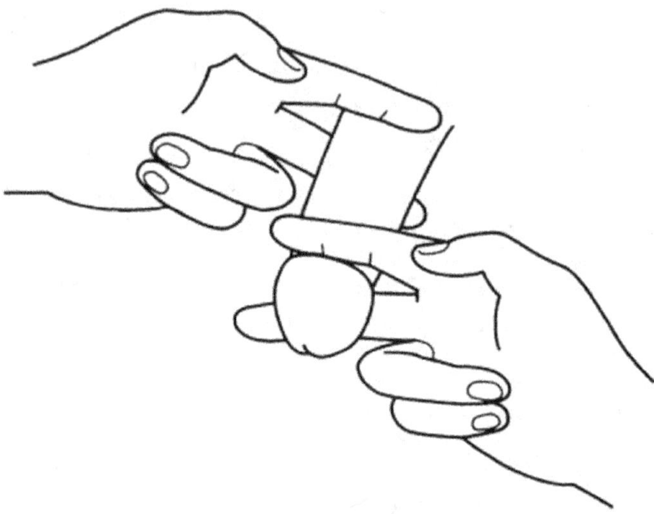

You certainly must maintain your vagina relaxed throughout the delicate penetration, otherwise it will be like attempting to push your lover through a locked door. That just won't work. When you penetrate the penis, it is most probable that you will want to peek between your legs at what you are doing, particularly at initially. You will accomplish this by elevating your upper body via clenching the abdominal muscles. As the belly tightens, so does the vagina and to prevent this tightness, direct your consciousness purposefully downward into the vagina in order to maintain it relaxed and open. I have discovered that reclining back for a bit, and intentionally relaxing my vagina once I get a hold of the penis and before insertion, allows me to broaden and relax the vaginal muscles. After you have done this, slide the soft penis in. As the penis and vagina relax, the simpler gentle penetration becomes. You may employ mild penetration as a technique of approaching lovemaking every time if you choose, or use it when you need it. But never forget.

A new sexual language

When you begin this new experience, it is crucial to remember to verbalize what you are experiencing. For instance, when a guy learns from his girlfriend that she can sense energy flowing from his soft, but unerect penis, it is a huge comfort. Learning that he is alive when soft is immensely comforting. He may stop thinking about erection and concentrate his concentration on the immediate sensation of the penis inside the vagina. This is a significantly more delicate level of experience and demands a calm of mind and an absence of nervous thoughts.

Putting the bodies together in this fashion is limited in excitement and opens up all sorts of additional possibilities for sexual interaction. Just leave it up to the genitals backed by your awareness, and they will perform whatever seems good to them. That is an entirely new sexual language. The penis may lay in the vagina, humming gently and pleasantly, or after a time it may start vibrating vigorously. It may get slowly and firmly erect, thrusting far up into the vagina, dancing and jerking upward, or relax down again, slithering all the way out, just to rise back up again in exhilarating penetration. With this union of opposites all sorts of wonders happen.

❧ Soft penetration is easy and a wonderful way to start making love.

❧ It means you can warm up together and be relaxed about it.

❧ "Share your now" to increase awareness and genital sensitivity.

❧ An erection can grow in response to the vagina, a thrilling sexual experience.

❧ Sexual energy arises from the interplay of male and female polarities.

CHAPTER THIRTEEN

DEEP PENETRATION

PENERATIONS OF WOMEN have failed to enjoy their heavenly orgasmic potential, the feminine thrill of sensuality and love via sex. The Garden of Love, the hidden entrance to sexual rapture for women and men, lies abandoned, unattended, and overrun with wandering weeds. All the emotional memories of a woman's unpleasant sexual experiences such as rape, abortion, aggressiveness, and abuse leave their psychological imprint in this deepest portion of the vagina. This induces constriction in the vaginal tissues, making the walls tight and inflexible.

In this manner, there is a continuing preventive barrier established in the tissues, and the vagina contracts reflexively during intercourse, restricting deeper entry. This implies that the strong positive penis head is unable to match easily and immediately with its negative counterpart in the deepest depths of the vagina, therefore disrupting the energy flow.

Women's sexual ecstasy

For a woman to feel these ecstatic energies in the depths of her vagina, the tensions and turbulence generated by previous occurrences must eventually be released so that the lady's negative pole becomes simple and innocent with a receptive receptivity. She is thus able to completely accept and use the beneficial masculine energy to flow inside her. The more sensitive the penis and vagina are to one other, and the longer a couple makes love in this trusting manner, the more it leads to an exquisite sensation of lovemaking. The energy exchange between the sexual organs is exhilarating enough to ground you firmly in the here and now, producing the dimension of Tantra quite organically.

Penetrate the depths and stay still

To reinforce the inherent nature of this polarity effect in our organs of love, they need to be intentionally healed and cleaned of poisonous tensions. This is done by deep, continuous penetration. For the woman, the focus location for healing is positioned deep at the apex of the vagina. It encompasses the sidewalls of the upper vaginal canal and up and around the cervix, which protrudes into this region of the vagina. This is her Garden of Love, the area where she will first discover genuine bliss in sex. When a woman is touched thus profoundly and deliberately by the penis, she may feel genuine love in her body via intercourse for the first time. A buddy experienced it as a pearl sliding up from the penis into her heart.

Here when she is a pure woman, her heart opens wonderfully and spontaneously, although it so seldom occurs. Instead, penetration is confined to brief thrusts concentrated on the first few centimeters of the vagina where many strong rings of muscle are discovered around the entrance. Friction-like quick motions back and forth at the entrance have the effect of causing extreme pleasure, which leads to excitation and consequently a desire for orgasm. With this, women's focus has been directed away from the knowledge of this gem in her upper vagina. Hardly has she had the chance to experience it with genuine sensitivity, and hence the wellspring of her true femininity remains untapped.

Women's (and men's) dependency on the clitoris for female orgasms has not improved things as far as vaginal awareness is concerned. Many women do not know the joy of a complete vaginal orgasm, and therefore for many of us, the clitoris becomes the major focus when making love. By performing vigorous thrusting pelvic motions focused on stimulating the clitoris, she can build the essential excitement for orgasm. Males too have gotten used to offering women sexual joy via the clitoris. The upshot of a lot of sexual excitation has been a relative desensitizing of the vagina. In the top section, she is protective, while in the bottom part, she is tight, tough, and eager.

Restoring masculine and feminine polarities

In its unparalleled wisdom, nature offers us the appropriate tool to fix the issue. Its strength is found in the potency of the penis. Deep, continuous penetration by the penis is the finest approach to restoring both the masculine and feminine polarity. Amazingly, the head of the penis behaves like a very sensitive magnet penetrating the energy field of the feminine pole. This has a significant impact on the stored vaginal tensions, prompting a discharge or dispersion experienced in a variety of ways, and in time the region is progressively modified to create lovely feminine energies. With this, both poles are reinforced. As a vital component of this healing process in the vagina, sensitivity and flexibility and awareness will also be restored to the penis itself. Males too have collected tensions and aches from misinterpretation, misuse, and abuse of their beautiful masculine antennae. This disruption has led to two major male extremes, one where there is too much tension in sex leading to premature ejaculation, and the other is impotence, a lack of responsiveness or sensitivity in the penis owing to sexual atrophy. Both these imbalances may be rectified by reducing the tensions collected in the male genitals.

Deep penetration is the method to touch the heavenly energies of a woman and for a man to realize his genuine sexual power. When a woman's body is properly prepared, her heart included, she becomes entirely sensuous, and will react spontaneously to love, which is extremely fulfilling to a man. Here lays his actual masculine power, to be unselfish enough to completely love a woman and give to her. The woman believes that her life has been enhanced energetically by being able to receive active energy, and the man becomes receptive by being able to offer, forming a circle in this exchange that fills us with the light of love.

Deep persistent penetration should be addressed as a technique of lovemaking, rather than something you perform rarely. Do so whenever it is feasible. A complete erection is essential and if the male discovers that he is not fully erect, he may use a little movement but he must avoid too much excitement. There should be just enough movement or excitement for a smooth, supple erection, not more. If the condition of erection occurs from mild penetration, then gently penetrate the depths of the vagina. To achieve this you may skillfully adjust the position by moving limbs around, if feasible without the penis losing touch with the vagina so that the male is then kneeling between the woman's knees. She lifts her knees to her chest and curls the pelvis upward to deepen or adjust the angle of the entry. Use some of the other Love Keys at the same time too, such as eyes meeting, breathing deeply and slowly, communication, and awareness in the

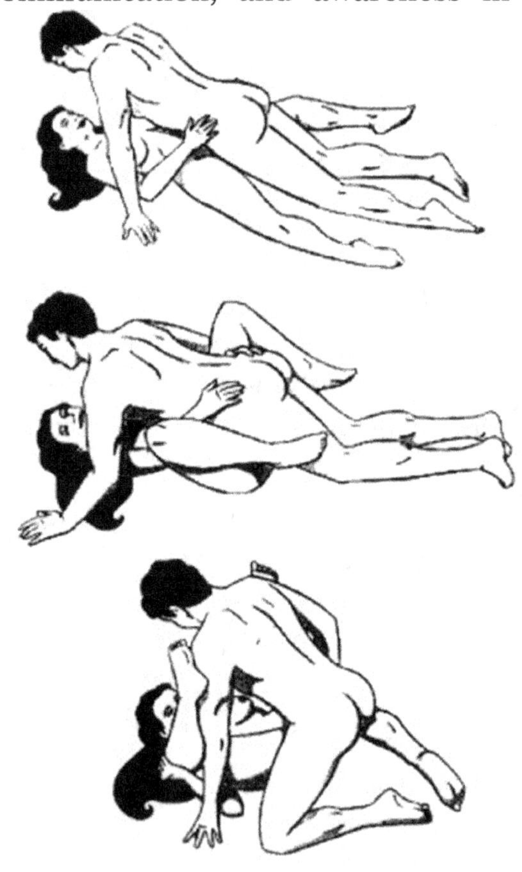

genitals (see fig. 10). Fig.10   Positions for deep sustained penetration

Slow and porous approach

Any hard thrust or insensitive approach will make the lady constrict her vagina in instinctive defense, so enter intentionally as gently as possible, millimeter by millimeter.

Go in as far as you can or until you feel some resistance against the head of your penis. You may be touching the cervix, the entry to the uterus, or the sides and upper borders of the vaginal canal. After you have got there, keep the penis motionless. Don't move. Keep your consciousness and concentration in the head of the penis, feeling from the root upward. Do not press up forcefully on the vaginal tissues; this is vital.

After you feel you have gone as deep as possible into the vagina, just draw back a hair's width. Truly as little as that! It makes all the difference, and will not harm your enjoyment in any way. Strangely, you are likely to feel more and not less. Let the contact between the penis and vagina be "porous", light, and airy. If you push up firmly you will compress the cells of the vagina, which will resist your incursion, pushing you away rather than welcoming you. A small piece of permeable space permits the male and female energies to interact, enabling the dispersing effect to take place. When this fraction of room is not granted, the sense is one of being crushed up against a wall.

Following a period of prolonged contact a pulse or throbbing may develop in the head of the penis at the spot where it is contacting the vaginal walls. When you sense this, stay calm and present for as long as you can, relaxing into the shifting feelings. Be with whatever is. It is excellent, over time, to open the vagina up from all sides; there is more room up and around the cervix, than we understand. To facilitate exploration of the untouched upper portions of the vagina, the male should shift his pelvis (and therefore the penis) gently to the side, to the right, or the left, and then keep still.

This is not to be misconstrued with a back-and-forth movement, rather it is a shift to the side wherein the male is shifting the angle of his pelvis, which then allows the penis to reach more distant locations. Then wait, allowing the intelligence of the penis to lead you. It may begin to move on its own, searching for areas of latent tension, or be deliciously sucked upward by the vagina. This magnetic brilliance is immensely affecting, a merging of man and woman, body and heart.

The lady should stay motionless and responsive, concentrating on her breasts and relaxing her vagina, retaining the awareness deep within where the penis is making contact. It will feel exhilarating, a heightened sensitivity, sometimes nearly overpowering, as a whole distinct sexual sensation unfolds. In the onset, the male may experience a shooting, buzzing, or electrical energy in his penis or through his body and he must stay here and now with this tremendous sense of pleasure.

That is a terrific pleasure, and the lady will also experience matching feelings, sometimes like calm waves of orgasm. Perhaps the entire region starts to glow golden, slowly growing in intensity, and spreading throughout the body. When you make love, keep exploring different positions which intensify penetration. To improve this exchange, picture your organs to be producers of love energy.

It may happen that after a period of this happy interaction, the penis abruptly starts to retreat and the male will begin to lose his erection. This may be quite worrisome, yet it is a process of nature, activity, and relaxation. After the penis has changed some energy it automatically settles into a calm condition. If a couple can continue to retain their awareness of the penis and vagina while this occurs, and stay still rather than move or lose interest, the penis will generally climb up again into the depths of the vagina.

Healing sexual pain and memories

At first, this purposeful touch via persistent deep penetration may likely feel harsh or painful in certain areas, and a woman could incline to withdraw away. It may also seem a little numb or distant, even deadened. It is crucial to note that the pain or numbness is typically reflecting some form of tension or cellular memory maintained in the tissue. Some women have felt pain reflecting the anus or the lower back, down the legs, and to locations where there may already be other health difficulties. The amount of pain, tension, and emotion present in a woman's vagina is strongly tied to her sexual history. Whatever degree of suffering or abuse we may have undergone, we all have our particular sexual history and its agonies resting exactly above our feminine pole.

These aches and memories are typically unconscious, and we are seldom aware of them. Yet when we slow down and bring mindfulness to treating the genitals, old emotional hurts buried in the past may arise. The first hint of pain or discomfort is not to be disregarded. Pain is an invitation, an indicator of tension; it suggests that a healing touch is required. The lady mustn't allow her boyfriend to push forcefully into this discomfort. We are not interested in adding agony to suffering; therefore allow him in just as deeply as seems comfortable to you.

Explain to him what is occurring to you. Rather than forcing him out, urging him to move back a bit, even a hair's width might be enough. Breathe, be interested, relax, and let the penis convert the agony.

Frequently the anguish will shift to strong pleasure or tears. This is a release of hidden emotional tension, which has generated hardness, and a lack of vaginal responsiveness. The tears, the agony, coughing, and any laughing that may occur apparently out of the blue are all signals that the vagina is softening and relaxing. If you are fortunate enough to experience this sort of release, you will feel an instant (and I mean immediate) alteration in the sensitivity of your vagina. Instantly your awareness is heightened as the pleasure and vigor of life seep throughout the surroundings. The guy too will sense a deep enlargement, a heightening of pleasure, and enhanced sensitivity in his penis.

In the same manner, a guy may also experience a spontaneous release of emotions, feel shooting pains, searing sensations, thankful tears of relief, and with it an instant strengthening of his real masculine vitality. If pain remains after the lovemaking it might imply an unexpressed emotional component, thus a guy is advised to enable himself to express his repressed sentiments. Using music to express the pain, finding a sound that vibrates from inside the suffering itself, and everything that comes from that expression, is one approach to relieve these tensions.

With this release of tensions via the persistent conscious presence of the penis in the vagina, a healing process is put into action. The penis heals and changes the vagina, and in so doing, the penis itself is healed and changed. It occurs as a result of its transformative force, and an intrinsic circle is completed, the penis and vagina are healed via each other; natural equilibrium is restored to man and woman. For such reasons, Tantra is regarded as a process of profound cleansing. We liberate the past by cleaning ourselves of its tensions, which constrain sexual energy and its wonderful growth. When the genitals become more pure, simple, and innocent, they can create sexual energy and this modifies the act. It becomes calm, motionless, and tranquil. Once the underlying magnetic intelligence is reintroduced to the sexual organs, it becomes a moving spiritual force, a happy inspiration. At last, we are able to touch and be touched by the other.

KEY POINTS:

- Male "positive" and female "negative" generate ecstatic streaming energies.
- Women's divine feminine energies are located in the upper part of the vagina.
- This ecstatic "Garden of Love" is to be consciously awakened by deep, sustained "porous" penetration.
- The head of the penis is similar to a powerful magnet.
- As the consciousness in the penis and vagina is purified, sexual ecstasy increases.
- Let sustained penetration be a "style" of lovemaking whenever erection is present.

CHAPTER FOURTEEN

ROTATING POSITION

Slow and porous approach

Any hard thrust or insensitive approach will make the lady constrict her vagina in instinctive defense, so enter intentionally as gently as possible, millimeter by millimeter. Go in as far as you can or until you feel some resistance against the head of your penis. You may be touching the cervix, the entry to the uterus, or the sides and upper borders of the vaginal canal. After you have got there, keep the penis motionless. Don't move. Keep your consciousness and concentration in the head of the penis, feeling from the root upward. Do not press up forcefully on the vaginal tissues; this is vital. After you feel you have gone as deep as possible into the vagina, just draw back a hair's width.

Truly as little as that! It makes all the difference, and will not harm your enjoyment in any way. Strangely, you are likely to feel more and not less. Let the contact between the penis and vagina be "porous", light, and airy. If you push up firmly you will compress the cells of the vagina, which will resist your incursion, pushing you away rather than welcoming you. A small piece of permeable space permits the male and female energies to interact, enabling the dispersing effect to take place. When this fraction of room is not granted, the sense is one of being crushed up against a wall.

Following a period of prolonged contact a pulse or throbbing may develop in the head of the penis at the spot where it is contacting the vaginal walls. When you sense this, stay calm and present for as long as you can, relaxing into the shifting feelings. Be with whatever is. It is excellent, over time, to open the vagina up from all sides; there is more room up and around the cervix, than we understand.

To facilitate exploration of the untouched upper portions of the vagina, the male should shift his pelvis (and therefore the penis) gently to the side, to the right, or the left, and then keep still. This is not to be misconstrued with a back-and-forth movement, rather it is a shift to the side wherein the male is shifting the angle of his pelvis, which then allows the penis to reach more distant locations. Then wait, allowing the intelligence of the penis to lead you. It may begin to move on its own, searching for areas of latent tension, or be deliciously sucked upward by the vagina. This magnetic brilliance is immensely affecting, a merging of man and woman, body and heart.

The lady should stay motionless and responsive, concentrating on her breasts and relaxing her vagina, retaining the awareness deep within where the penis is making contact. It will feel exhilarating, a heightened sensitivity, sometimes nearly overpowering, as a whole distinct sexual sensation unfolds. In the onset, the male may experience a shooting, buzzing, or electrical energy in his penis or through his body and he must stay here and now with this tremendous sense of pleasure.

That is a terrific pleasure, and the lady will also experience matching feelings, sometimes like calm waves of orgasm. Perhaps the entire region starts to glow golden, slowly growing in intensity, and spreading throughout the body. When you make love, keep exploring different positions which intensify penetration. To improve this exchange, picture your organs to be producers of love energy.

It may happen that after a period of this happy interaction, the penis abruptly starts to retreat and the male will begin to lose his erection. This may be quite worrisome, yet it is a process of nature, activity, and relaxation. After the penis has changed some energy it automatically settles into a calm condition. If a couple can continue to retain their awareness of the penis and vagina while this occurs, and stay still rather than move or lose interest, the penis will generally climb up again into the depths of the vagina.

Healing sexual pain and memories

At first, this purposeful touch via persistent deep penetration may likely feel harsh or painful in certain areas, and a woman could incline to withdraw away. It may also seem a little numb or distant, even deadened. It is crucial to note that the pain or numbness is typically reflecting some form of tension or cellular memory maintained in the tissue. Some women have felt pain reflecting the anus or the lower back, down the legs, and to locations where there may already be other health difficulties. The amount of pain, tension, and emotion present in a woman's vagina is strongly tied to her sexual history. Whatever degree of suffering or abuse we may have undergone, we all have our particular sexual history and its agonies resting exactly above our feminine pole.

These aches and memories are typically unconscious, and we are seldom aware of them. Yet when we slow down and bring mindfulness to treating the genitals, old emotional hurts buried in the past may arise. The first hint of pain or discomfort is not to be disregarded. Pain is an invitation, an indicator of tension; it suggests that a healing touch is required. The lady mustn't allow her boyfriend to push forcefully into this discomfort. We are not interested in adding agony to suffering; therefore allow him in just as deeply as seems comfortable to you.

Explain to him what is occurring to you. Rather than forcing him out, urging him to move back a bit, even a hair's width might be enough. Breathe, be interested, relax, and let the penis convert the agony.

Frequently the anguish will shift to strong pleasure or tears. This is a release of hidden emotional tension, which has generated hardness, and a lack of vaginal responsiveness. The tears, the agony, coughing, and any laughing that may occur apparently out of the blue are all signals that the vagina is softening and relaxing. If you are fortunate enough to experience this sort of release, you will feel an instant (and I mean immediate) alteration in the sensitivity of your vagina. Instantly your awareness is heightened as the pleasure and vigor of life seep throughout the surroundings. The guy too will sense a deep enlargement, a heightening of pleasure, and enhanced sensitivity in his penis.

In the same manner, a guy may also experience a spontaneous release of emotions, feel shooting pains, searing sensations, thankful tears of relief, and with it an instant strengthening of his real masculine vitality. If pain remains after the lovemaking it might imply an unexpressed emotional component, thus a guy is advised to enable himself to express his repressed sentiments. Using music to express the pain, finding a sound that vibrates from inside the suffering itself, and everything that comes from that expression, is one approach to relieve these tensions.

With this release of tensions via the persistent conscious presence of the penis in the vagina, a healing process is put into action. The penis heals and changes the vagina, and in so doing, the penis itself is healed and changed. It occurs as a result of its transformative force, and an intrinsic circle is completed, the penis and vagina are healed via each other; natural equilibrium is restored to man and woman. For such reasons, Tantra is regarded as a process of profound cleansing. We liberate the past by cleaning ourselves of its tensions, which constrain sexual energy and its wonderful growth. When the genitals become purer, the position itself is irrelevant in tantric sex; what counts is who occupies the position.

As a result, because individuals create the postures, there are no positions that are specifically defined for Tantra. Your goal should be to make the job successful. Almost any position will be ideal for you if you're calm, at the moment, and breathing normally, but to change your sexual reality, you must be fully inside of yourself. The sense of life inside the body is the Tantric sexual presence.

Genital communion

Every position's primary goal should be to improve genital communion by increasing the depth and contact between the penis and vagina. Also, it ought to be cozy. Otherwise, when the body is under stress, consciousness is diverted. The posture you choose should heighten the sensation, which might be tingling, flowing, a sense of electrical exchange, or anything else that could be present. We may now change the way we generally think about sex positions and movement because of our new knowledge of the penis and vagina as complimentary poles and two components of one entity. To maximize the energy potential, it is quite beneficial if they fit tightly together. The touch becomes much more sensuous when a lady spreads her labia wide after (or before) entrance.

Remember that pressing too firmly against the vaginal walls will nullify this magnetic sensitivity as you penetrate as deeply as you can while allowing for a "porous" touch. In Tantra, the goal is to maintain the penis and vagina as an immobile focus point while allowing the bodies to stay together or move as a single unit. The bodies themselves choose inventive postures to accommodate the genital connection when we keep this in mind.

Regular sex involves pushing and pulling away from one another while simultaneously pushing toward each other with pelvic thrusting motions. You move back and forth, driving the penis into and out of the vagina without giving them any opportunity to communicate. But, in Tantra, the penis does not exit the vagina when you move as a unit. The bodies rotate and move around this basic link, which remains completely inside the vagina (see fig. 11), with each position facilitating the sexual interaction. This rhythm of thrusting and friction-like motions in sex is quickly replaced by the excitement of these spinning alterations in position.

Moreover, males will discover that some pleasurable movement is possible within the vagina without really moving out or causing any friction. His penis will start to guide him in how to make love as he develops in sensitivity and stillness, telling him when to move or change positions and when to remain motionless or probing. The male gives his penis power and faith, which elevates the act of making love into a celestial experience.

Experimenting with rotating positions, keeping your awareness

Sexual energy will continue to change and move since it is a dynamic, living force that is in no way static. As a result, you must pay close attention to what is going on between the genitalia when moving and modifying your body. Spin around the genital connection and you'll discover that if you start, for example, in the scissors position mentioned for mild penetration, a fascinating series of rotating positions is conceivable.

Any number of roles may be readily discovered without having to be very creative. In actuality, your body arranges into a new posture with every centimeter you move.

Try it out for yourself to see how easily the bodies can roll about in unison. You may first investigate options without penetrating. Imagine that your genitalia is linked while you lie on a carpeted floor together in any position.

A series of postures will then start to take shape as you move the bodies in synchrony while maintaining the pelvises firmly joined (to prevent the penis from leaving the vagina). Maintain each posture for a little while before shifting again. The body can find the ideal posture for the situation, whether it is for a second or an hour, with this flexibility and choice. You can support this connection between the poles and the flow of energy with your bodies if you keep your focus there. The two bodies may combine into a fluid ball of energy that rolls about with its velocity when they are properly, and innocent, they can create sexual energy and this modifies the act. It becomes calm, motionless, and tranquil. Once the underlying magnetic intelligence is reintroduced to the sexual organs, it becomes a moving spiritual force, a happy inspiration. At last, we can touch and be touched by the other proportioned.

Fig. 11   Sequence of rotating positions through front

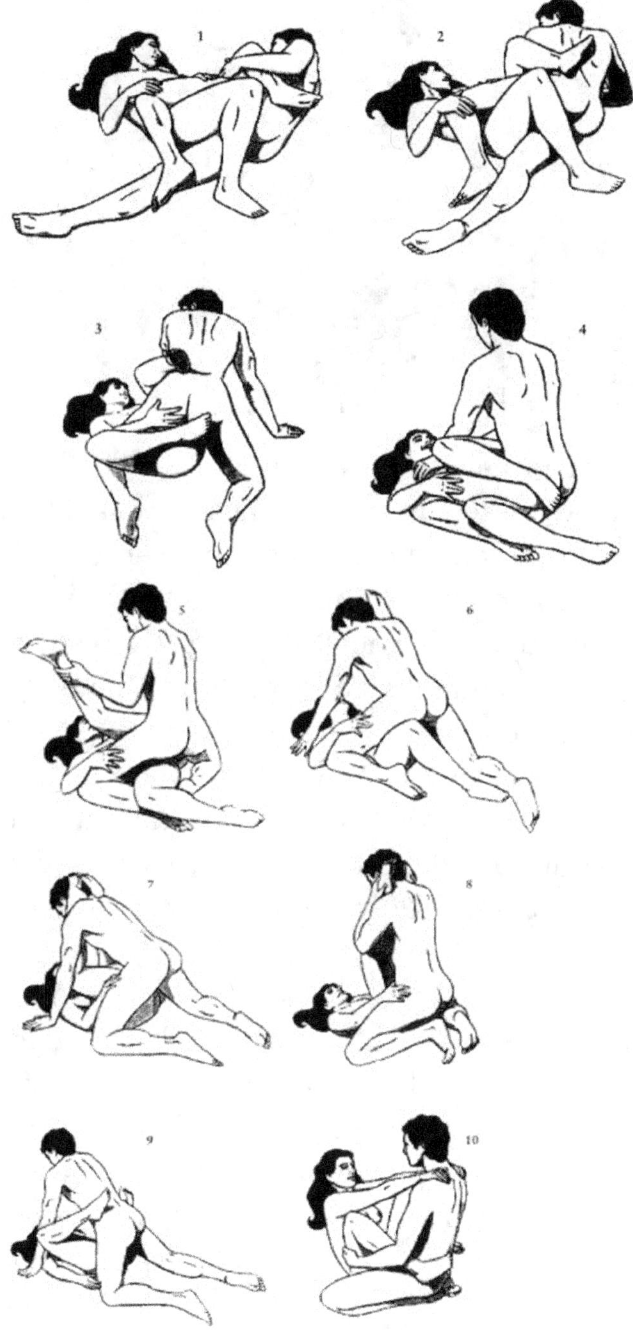

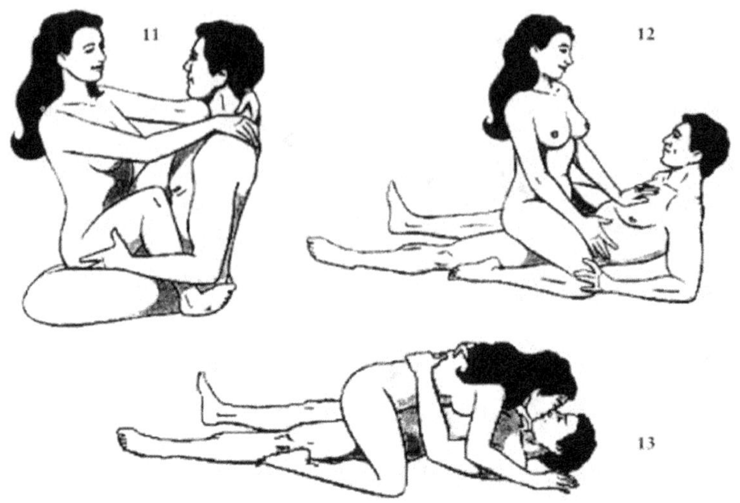

Changing position creates a presence

The location of the mind matters more than the position of the body when you concentrate on awareness and presence. You could then wish to adjust your positions if you change your mind. Thus, armed with this new knowledge, start to respect and trust your body's wisdom and give it space. Let the body act on a natural inclination rather than fighting it. If you suddenly feel the want to make love on top but a voice within your head warns you that you once tried it and it caused him to lose his erection, go ahead and try it. Put the past's whispers away and give in to the present. Do your best to stay present oneself.

When the body positions itself in a way that makes you feel open and defenseless, it signals that you are "here," that something is new and uncharted. Spend some time in this position. Keep in mind that this is the intensity of the current moment rather than attempting to leave it to lessen your misery. In the same manner, alter your posture if you catch yourself daydreaming or feeling drowsy and absent. This changes the genital connection right away and gives you your presence back.

You will discover that, at least initially, your old favorite positions no longer help you in your new orientation once you start to grasp how sexual energy reacts best. For instance, if he has always pushed his pelvis from this posture in the past, the guy on top will probably feel a tremendous amount of pressure to act. When your body and mind are itching to "do" something, it might initially be challenging to "be" in a position.

The lady may take the dominant role so that the male can unwind more readily. It took me some time to relax into "being" when I first tried this because as soon as I was in the lead, I felt like I had to contribute as well. I could easily feel awkward, unnatural, or under pressure. Yet, I have also discovered that when I am in a real sexual flow, my body and my partner's body will naturally assume the required posture.

Given this, there are many postures that two bodies may assume, so use your imagination and keep switching things up (see fig. 12). You can do this without disconnecting, but keep in mind to rotate around the genitalia. If the penis accidentally pops out of the vagina, just put it back in and find a comfortable position. People in relationships may sometimes tell me, "This posture works for me but not for him, thus we are having troubles." I remind them that the penis and vagina work as a single unit to perform sexual acts. So, if a stance is ineffective for one partner, it is also ineffective for the other. It's preferable to give up that stance and consider other ones. I also mention how the bodies become softer, more flexible, and less scared the more times couples make love when they are unwinding. They often discover that once challenging jobs are now simple.

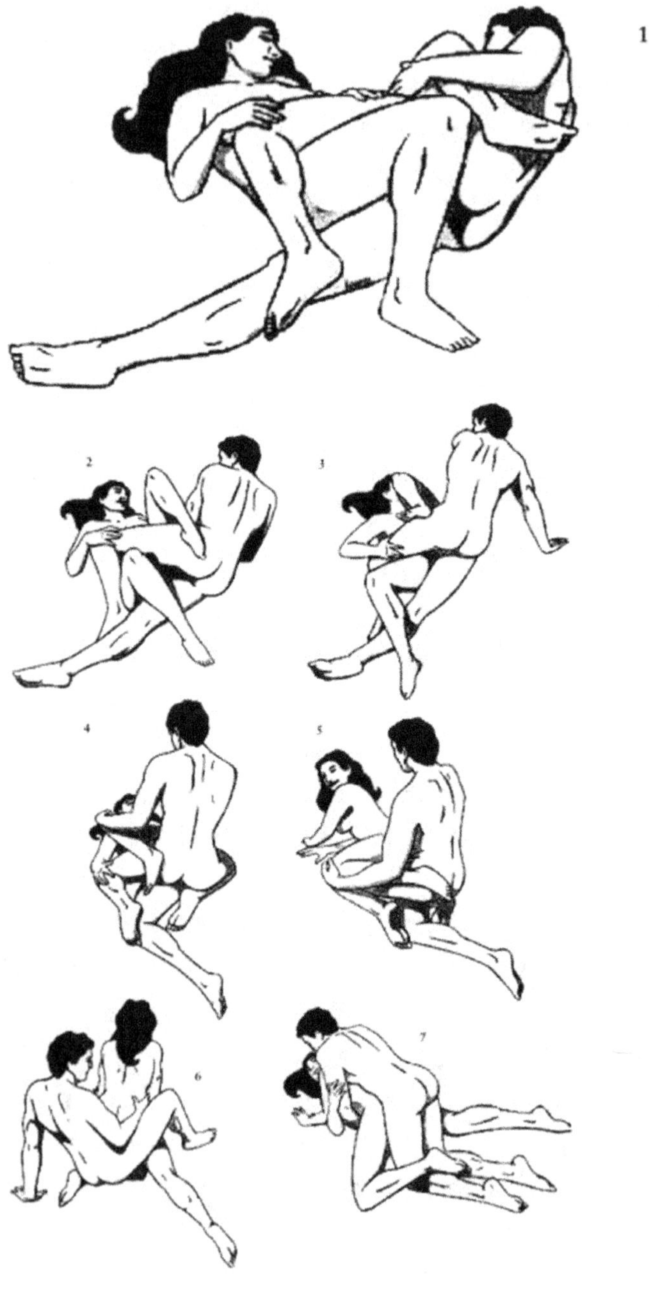

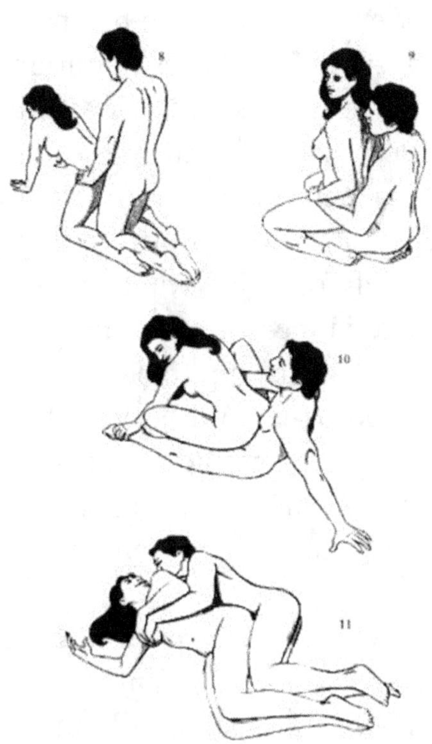

Staying conscious in exploration

It is crucial to understand that certain stances are inherently harmful. You could slip into them because it seems comfortable to revert to previous excitement habits, but they won't be very rewarding. When I first started practicing Tantra, I discovered that anytime I was pierced from behind, doggy style, I would get so excited that I would lose consciousness. I quickly discovered that rather than my body, it was mostly occurring in my thoughts. I can appreciate that position once again without getting caught up in excitement or imagination now that my presence and sexual awareness are so much stronger.

To remain enigmatic here and now while taking in the pulsating masculine energy, however, requires continual awareness. I often decided to let go of awareness and joyfully and carelessly ride the thrill ride of excitement while having a great time. Yet with time, I discovered that the exhilaration from earlier paled in comparison to the ecstasy of being present and in genital communion when in that specific posture and with that specific angle of entry.

The most interesting part of discovering sex is probably this. Making love continuously while slowly realizing what's going on and piecing together a new image is incredibly wonderful. The intensity rises as various emotions begin to leave the body, and you feel more receptive and open, and because the emotions appear in response to love, profound healing is possible. Love can erase the hurts of the past, sometimes through laughter, sometimes through quiet, and sometimes through tears.

Certain postures are just naturally cozy, which promotes prolonged passionate encounters. Sometimes, it's fantastic to just plug in, shut your eyes, lean back, and spend an hour or two in complete awareness (see fig. 13).

Because of its relative neutrality, the scissors position—which involves the male laying on his side, the woman resting on her back, opening her legs, and bringing her pelvis to his—is an excellent choice for delicate penetration. No one is on top or below; it is well-balanced and, more importantly, cozy for both. Also, it's easy for most individuals to locate, making it a comfortable position to begin making out.

The traditional "doing" or missionary position, the man on top (see fig. 14), may be utilized well for both "non-doing" and deep penetration. The penetration is kept deep and motionless by the guy just lying forward or kneeling over the lady. To help in penetration, the lady might lift her legs and curve her pelvis upward. From this position, rolling to one side or the other while keeping close contact with the vagina is simple. The pair faces each other on their sides as the male rests between the woman's legs, using cushions to make the position comfortable. These postures are especially beneficial for genital cleaning and healing, which call for deep penetration.

Fig. 13   Side position: relaxed and serene with eyes closed

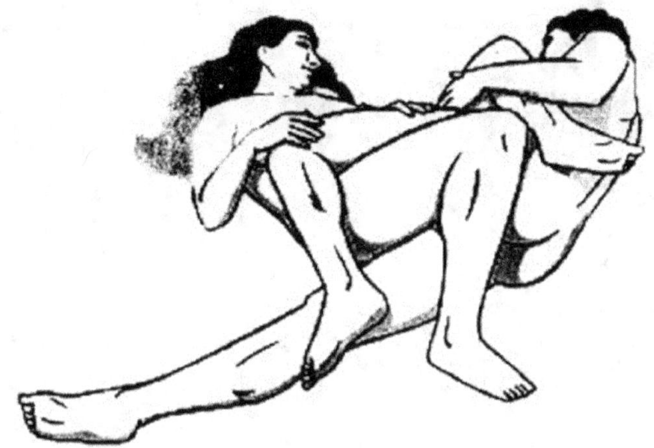

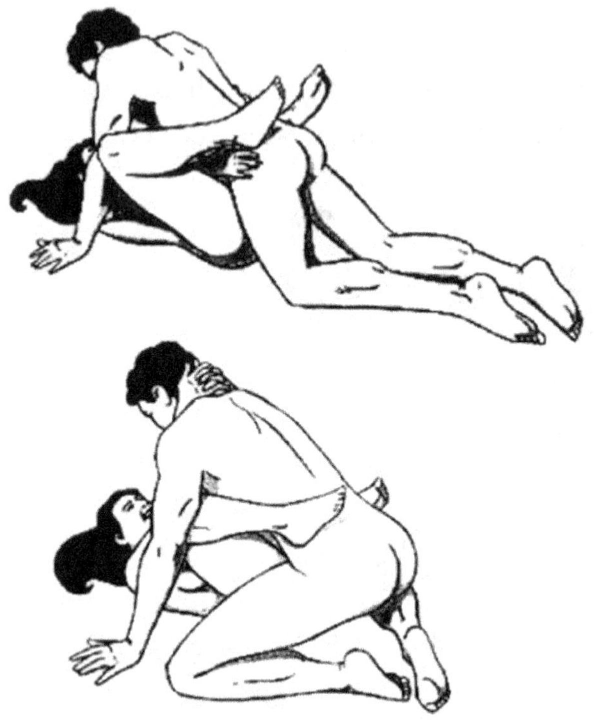

Fig. 14   Man on top position

The Yab Yum position—an ecstatic circle of energy

The spine and body energy are upright in the sitting posture, also known as the Yab Yum position (see fig. 15), which has the benefits of gravitational levitation and alignment with heaven and earth. Here, the lips, eyes, and chest easily converge, creating an ecstatically satisfying circle of energy between the bodies. To make it simpler for you both to hold this position while trying it out, place a cushion beneath the woman's buttocks. This will support her pelvis and help you both feel more comfortable. Just act if it seems good to you. When the sexual channels are open, the sexual energy will naturally arrange the body in certain postures based on the energetic force between the bodies, rather than as a result of a deliberate choice.

There are sex manuals that outline certain postures that are thought to have a magical effect, but they came from the wisdom of two aware bodies, not the mind, as is sometimes claimed. These postures become empty shells with no inherent worth when they are transformed into procedures that are not supported by the awareness and sexual energy. In this case, particular positions are not a concern. Instead, adopt the Yab Yum posture, focusing on your genitalia while you make love. Whenever you feel drowsy or insensitive, switch positions, and you'll discover that you're instantly more conscious of the sexual energy. The postures will be taken care of when you let the bodies react to one another and dance together.

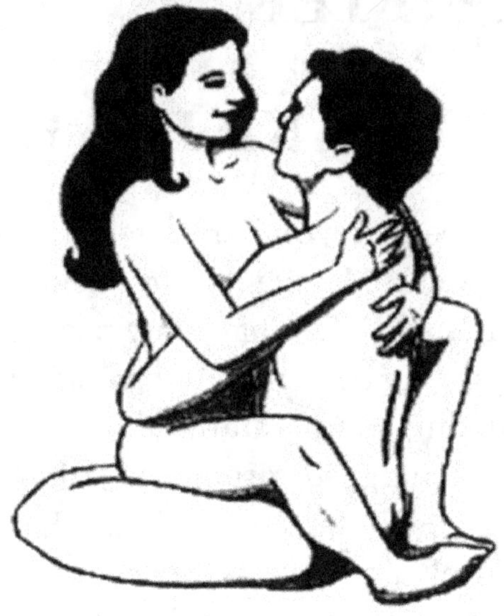

Fig. 15   Yab Yum position

- Presence and awareness are more important than positions.
- The vagina and the penis within it form one unit.
- Preserve this unity to increase the possibility of energetic exchange.
- Change positions by rotating around the genital connection.
- This naturally changes the angle of penetration to increase sensitivity.
- Shifting positions bring presence, life, and dance into love.

CHAPTER FIFTEEN

MAKE A DATE TO MAKE LOVE

Often, we schedule business meetings, dinner dates, and theater dates instead of romantic ones. Making love frequently comes in last on the list, even though it is what most people think about most. The majority of us contemplate love after finishing our job, eating, drinking, and entertaining. We decide to make love when we are fatigued, drunk, have just finished a large meal, or all three of these. To anticipate that such an encounter would be a lovely and reverent celebration of love is unreasonable, if not unjust, given that this is rarely the moment when we are at our finest.

Making plans to go out to supper or the movies is often done to return home and go to bed. But, we are seated, our legs crossed and uncrossed, devouring course after course of talk while tensely wondering when or if it will ever happen! Yet, once I had the guts to be open and honest with a guy about what I wanted, I felt immediate relief, my energy could flow freely, and this enabled me to be natural.

I've always enjoyed it when a guy is forward about his desires when he speaks out and tells me he wants to make love without the customary game that comes before sex. In modern culture, it's unusual to go on a date only to make out. Yet, many couples who have used this strategy claim that initially there was resistance since it eliminated the spontaneity of sex, but they eventually reported that it worked out extremely well. The ladies said that once they let go of the notion that they were "making love on demand," knowing that they would undoubtedly make love with their spouse offered them great satisfaction.

More open and accessible, they felt more valued and liked. When they were aware that they would be having sex at a certain time, the males claimed to feel a great deal more at ease since their sex-related mental fixation decreased. Without persistent sexual ideas or fears, many discovered it was simpler to focus on other tasks throughout the day. Several said that knowing they had a planned date to have sexual relations prevented them from compulsively staring at other women.

The fact is that spontaneity seldom occurs, despite what individuals claim they desire. We repeatedly engage in the same behavior in sex. The question of whether and when women will allow them to have another sexual encounter worries males a lot. We've all heard jokes about how women have a habit of getting headaches at night, and they have been known to purposefully avoid having sex with their spouses. The guy is agitated and worried, wondering when she would allow him to enter her again. The male finds comfort in knowing that she will be there, prepared and eager to make love. He feels at ease because he is aware that he won't have to convince her or win her over.

As a result, he gains a natural loving authority that enables him to channel his masculine energy creatively. Thus it becomes crucial that the woman doesn't invent justifications when it's time to make love. While there will undoubtedly be times when she is unable to engage for actual reasons, making love is often beneficial and very engaging regardless of what else is going on. In addition to benefiting the woman, the male also benefits when the woman follows through on her promise to make love. Knowing that love will happen may also help to delay the making of love since fear would lead to tension, which would then lead to excitement and a higher chance of early ejaculation.

Without a partner or prior planning, making out in public suggests that less thought is put into the act. I discovered that being aware of the outcome beforehand made me a more sensitive lover when I started going on dates to make love. A few hours before the event, I could tune into sex and become aware of my breasts and vagina, which let me ingest the awareness before my partner showed up. I was nearly ready to be penetrated when we eventually laid down together. The thought of working together in this fashion, as well as the mental preparation that goes along with it, alters the whole nature of romantic love.

Sexual Dating

It's probable that when you first begin "dating" in this manner, you first feel a bit uncomfortable, even bashful or uneasy, particularly when it's time to get dressed and go to bed. It may be difficult in and of itself to decide to do this rather than

you make love intentionally, no energy is lost or squandered. You will be producing energy, and you will feel energized. You could even notice that you start to need less sleep.

I advise giving yourself at least two to three hours on your date when you want to make love. Lock the door and turn on the answering machine to make sure there are no interruptions. Lack of privacy may cause worries that can lead to sexual desire and make it hard to relax during the experience. If at all possible, avoid just making love at night; instead, pick out moments when your body is awake and alert, perhaps after some dancing, yoga, or meditation. To find out what works best for you, try dates at various times of the day. Since the day has barely begun, mornings are ideal. After a good night's sleep, the body is refreshed and the mind is mostly quiet and free of the worries of the day. Many couples also like the afternoons, so if your job schedule prevents it, try the weekends instead.

Even if it means leaving your kids with friends for the day, you must attempt it. then make love rather than watch a movie! After a two-hour conversation with me, one couple decided to start spending Friday mornings together several years ago. To have some time at home while the kids were in school, they adjusted their work schedules. Even the neighbors were aware of the beautiful silence in the area around the home as it became a holy day. This weekly date greatly aided their relationship, and the children also benefitted from the joyful atmosphere that their parents' intentional love created for them.

Love in the center of your life

Not that you have to wait till you have two or three hours to make love. Tantra offers a version of the sexual "quickie" that focuses more on plugging in than going for it when there isn't much time to make love. Just insert the relaxed penis into the vagina as advised in the section on mild penetration, and then layered together in awareness for 20 minutes. It might infuse your day with a new air of happiness if you join in like way in the morning after coffee and before work.

Try fifteen minutes of energy exchange as a goodnight kiss if you're drowsy but still feel the need to be close to your partner. Even better, you may doze off in this manner while the darkness falls cheerfully about you. Make a date to make love before you go if you are parting ways with your partner for a while; even 10 minutes may be magical. It is lovely to bid someone farewell in a thoughtful manner as opposed to saying your goodbyes in a hurried or emotional embrace at an airport gate.

You may put love back at the center of your life by setting up a date to make love. When making small conversation with friends suddenly doesn't appeal to you as much and you're eager to go home and joyfully collapse into bed with your partner, there is a lot less time spent. Some couples, especially those who have been together for a long time, have found it necessary to arrange a time for romantic intimacy, fitting it around the demands of their kids, their in-laws, and their peers.

During the weekends, they gather in a circle and schedule meetings! Never be intimidated by the thought of working for two to three hours. Make it open-ended so that you won't have to worry about the conclusion; that's what's crucial. There is no doubt that you must come to the present and be there for the whole 128 minutes. Have a hot bath together, dance, give each other massages, make out, have a cup of tea, and then make out again. A little pause is usually a good idea if it appears like nothing is occurring. Usually, it has a wonderful effect on both of you, renewing you, and when you restart, it's a brand-new experience. Making a date to make love in this manner, whether it lasts for a long time or is brief, can assist to refocus your relationship. Many couples find that making love whenever they can is important, and they quickly learn that sexual chemistry is the foundation of their relationships. Your personal experience becomes more profound the more often you make love. Also, it gives the body a very beneficial dose of quiet, and even daily tasks take on a more concentrated character.

The enormous strain of expectations we have about the sexual act, which obstructs our ability to be present, is also lessened by this frequency. If we make love regularly, it is much simpler for us to "be." Whatever occurs will happen because we are at ease and ease. Exploration and discovery are possible with this unassuming approach.

Create an atmosphere of intimacy

You may need some alone time to discuss, to express your thoughts about the day's events or any ambiguous emotions you are having. When you start making out with your partner, make sure that they are out in the open. If you don't, your unsaid worries and fears will keep you from enjoying the moment. Particularly when they go unspoken, your sentiments might serve as a subtle barrier limiting greater energy connection between you and your partner. While the intellect struggles mightily to find excuses not to express its emotions, sexual energy responds to candor.

Psychological openness has been linked to higher levels of physical enjoyment, according to several couples. Tantra cautions us to engage in sexual activity only when we are feeling loving and generous and advises against using sex to bind us together if we are even somewhat irritable. Once your return to earth, it is best to unwind and massage each other as you both become clear and calm and rekindle your closeness. Next, have a love affair much, much later.

The Love Keys may be used to experiment when you go on a date to make love, and you now have a range of ideas to test out. You should start experimenting with everything you can recall. Nevertheless, your key is whatever works for you. It may not be one of the recommendations listed here, but if it makes it easier for you to be more mindful, it is the key. Breathing, maintaining eye contact, being aware of the positive polarity, and resting your feet are just a few of the keys you may utilize at once. There are an unlimited number of keys to assist with internal awareness change, and as your sensitivity increases, the keys grow softer.

KEY POINTS:

- Agreeing on a time to make love puts love back in your life.

- It increases relaxation, consciousness, and commitment.

- Each meeting is an opportunity to experiment with the Love Keys.

- The more we make love, the more we wish to make love.

- The well-used words "making love" regain their original meaning as we feel the influence of love in our lives.

CHAPTER SIXTEEN

FOREPLAY AFRESH

So that our energies may awaken and gradually attune to one another, WARMING UP TO LOVEMAKING is crucial. The difference is that it enables space for a spontaneous attraction to develop. Both men and women benefit from it, while women do so more so. Women require and value the moment before penetration because they are the negative polarity, and they want this time to be completely open to love. Also, it must be a loving and kind game rather than a serious endeavor with predetermined objectives carried out as if following a mechanical handbook.

Foreplay's most important quality in a novel approach to intimacy is that it shouldn't be too exciting. While it may be tempting at times, avoid making your spouse too enthusiastic. Moving into a peaceful sexual encounter is challenging because of this. Sexual stimulation may arouse lust or arouse desire, which releases energy. Because of this, it will be challenging to remain awake and aware of the present. The attitude of the mind is the most crucial component of the Tantric method of foreplay.

The important part is how you do something, not what you do. A certain mindset, method, and goal are needed if you want to make your spouse hot and horny. Everything will change depending on where and how you touch. Yet a guy who invests the time to slowly and sensually approach a lady and softly arouse her body will experience the welcoming atmosphere after penetration has taken place.

Rediscovering erogenous zones

Erogenous zones were created by nature and work in a way that stimulates and arouses sexual desire. The buzzing of the life force itself might be sensed as excitement, which shouldn't be mistaken with excitement. These erogenous zones serve as portals to the present and aid us in gaining access to our life force.

Unfortunately, because of our ignorance of sex, we often misuse or abuse our erogenous areas, which causes them to eventually lose their sensitivity. This may manifest as insensitivity, where we physically retreat from the other and hence from ourselves, or it may seem as hypersensitivity, where we become intolerably sensitive and even repulsed by contact. It's possible for the body to feel leaden, numb, or lifeless.

Women's nipples, for instance, may go from being dull and unresponsive to being painfully sensitive to contact. Either response has the propensity to drive the other person away right away. The clitoris is also susceptible to harm, particularly if it is often utilized for orgasm. A lady may become sexually withdrawn just as her lover is attempting to touch her because of an insensitive touch that has a repulsive impact.

Tantra teaches us that a woman's positive pole and the entrance to her sexual expression are her breasts and nipples and that they may carry her to the depths and peaks of ecstasy. Her feminine sexual energy travels via her breasts. So, a woman's ability to be sensitive and to embrace and receive care for her breasts takes on more significance. A guy must be careful how he touches her because he wants her to respond and open up to the contact rather than react to it.

A helpful rule of thumb is to observe how the approach affects your body's energy and note if it causes more excitement and tension or greater inner sensitivity and expansion. It is lovely and natural for a woman to touch her penis, but often she wants it to be erect right away so that penetration and pleasure may occur. Using friction by sliding the hand back and forth is the traditional method for starting an erection. It will be more challenging for the guy to enter the lady gently and mindfully if he experiences this sort of stimulation, which will make him eager, restless, and impatient.

By performing motions analogous to masturbating, the penis senses an unsaid pressure and need for an erection, which may sometimes make it more challenging for him to get. After a guy is within a woman, he will then need to continually maintain and build up the degree of sexual arousal to stay erect since this form of erection, which depends on stimulation, may be temperamental, delicate, and quick to lose. This may cause intercourse to become frantic and overexcited, which causes ejaculation to occur quickly.

This may be a lovely experience, a fantastic exchange of energy, where the penis is fondled and massaged leisurely without the purpose to induce an erection if the touch is kind and not demanding. When the woman just touches the penis with her loving presence, when she rubs, squeezes, or pulls the folds of the foreskin back, the penis will absorb the love, sense the interest, and react appropriately. The erection will be a byproduct of the love, and it will be of a different quality than when it results from mental or physical stress. The goal is to admire and cherish the penis for all of its great features as a powerful instrument for love and healing. The penis notices the shift in the woman's attitude and feels more in control.

Relax to expand energy and extend your lovemaking

Playing with excitement is a normal occurrence and lovely energy; however, just use a little amount of it to get you warmed up and start a fire before relaxing into the fun of it. Tantric and conventional sex both start with a craving for some life and a spark of attraction. Tantra, however, sticks with the beginning, therefore the similarities stop at this point. If you want, you could let it go on for hours. The fire we lit will soon turn into fading embers in traditional sex, where anticipation is built up. For many individuals, sex only lasts a few minutes because of how quickly the wind rushes through and burns the fire.

Tantra forbids activities that fan the flame and make it burn too rapidly. As an alternative, we remain amid the original attraction's flames and fan them with knowledge and presence. The body will eventually be consumed by the fire, which will keep it brilliant and blazing for hours. Maintaining your awareness of the demands of each moment while feeling as if you are floating underneath the energy. If a little excitement is required to keep the erection, try to get yourself going for a short period, possibly by moving. After that, unwind once more while maintaining your composure and continuing to make love until you feel deeply satisfied. When a couple can have this sort of sexual connection, they discover that they are more in love with one another and that collaboration comes naturally to them in everyday life.

While you touch and caress your lover, pay attention to how they react. Avoid going to locations that may thrill your partner excessively, or try touching the same spot differently. It is preferable to do something gentle and acknowledging rather than aggressive since the vagina and clitoris have long been and incorrectly been the focus of arousing attention during foreplay. For instance, the clitoris produces a considerable quantity of excitation when rubbed quickly. Try only touching it with your fingertips, without doing anything else. Move your finger slowly if you must. Another option is to softly cup your whole palm over your pubic bone and keep it there motionless for many minutes. Spread love and positive energy via your hand.

A pleasant turn-on may be achieved by lightly stroking, tugging, and playing with the pubic hair, or by lightly tapping the pubic bone. In general, a gentle, caring touch increases bodily energy and increases sensitivity; it is an immediate turn-on. In contrast, forced or abrasive, demanding contact leads the body to constrict and harden in defense, decreasing receptivity.

Oral sex in foreplay

You may be wondering at this point about the benefits of oral sex during foreplay. It has become a crucial component of sexual activity for many individuals, but its euphoric potential is unknown since the engagement of the penis in the vagina alone does not satisfy profoundly. Oral stimulation of the penis and clitoris, on the other hand, results in intense excitation and lowers genital awareness. Oral sex, according to both men and women, desensitizes the penis and vagina and nullifies the dramatic consequences of straightforward conscious penetration.

We can now see that there is almost no bio-electric alignment between the mouth and the genitalia thanks to our knowledge of polarity, both positive and negative. Although oral sex may be thrilling, the deeper energies are not aroused, and after tasting the blissful magnetic function of the penis and vagina, oral sex might gradually lose its appeal or be sometimes enjoyed for amusement.

For women, the topic of lubrication comes up during foreplay. If we are avoiding stimulation of any type, it is preferable to utilize lubricant or saliva instead of lubrication, which is often acquired with some kind of stimulation. Put a little amount at the vaginal opening before moving on to the penis. Don't be ashamed to recommend spreading it on slowly and sensually from the head to the root since it may be enjoyable and counts as foreplay. Guys are more than happy to utilize it since it makes it easy for them to easily glide inside the lady, and they like doing so! Keep in mind to apply it so that the penis feels alive rather than hungry. Not agitating but lubricating is the goal.

A woman may discover that her vagina lubricates itself more readily after having love calmly. Less stimulation is needed when the vagina and its surrounding tissues relax and become more sensitive and receptive. Just a tiny quantity of lubrication is required here and on the head of the penis to ease entrance since a relaxed vagina is generally smooth and moist.

Touching breasts and chest

Most women want to touch and love their breasts because it combines their upper and bottom bodies and leads to a profound sexual delight. When the breasts are caressed, warmth and life flow into the vagina. On the other hand, a woman may get quickly agitated or excited when her breasts are tightly pinched or overstimulated, which may encourage her to orgasm. She could be pushed to the brink by this, going from sensation to hysteria in a matter of seconds! In this instance, the nipples' response is not a genuine one; rather, it is a conditioned response that gives rise to sexual tension, passion, and anticipation. The natural reaction of the breasts and nipples expands the body's energy, softens the heart, and pours an abundance of warm vitality into the vagina. It doesn't have anything to do with obtaining anything; instead, it helps you become more present, enthusiastic, and engaged at the moment.

This will be quite helpful for both of you if you instruct your partner on how to touch your breasts and nipples. When a guy touches a woman's breasts, she should encourage him to do so in a manner that will allow her to take in and process his touch. Her heart will be more vulnerable and her sexual energy will be more intense the more deeply she feels. It is very advised that a woman start her breast awareness cultivation so that she is not only dependent on her spouse to awaken her positive pole. She is urged to "hold" her breasts at the forefront of her consciousness during lovemaking and other times (both nipples at once), filling them with energy, and melting into them to ignite her body electricity. And to further this knowledge, a lady might touch her breasts while in a sexual act.

Many guys also have sensitive nipples, where they want to be caressed. Include the whole chest and heart region in your caress as you do so. When you do so, stroke the chest to feel its hairy or silky muscle textures. Consider applying pressure to the "Love Spot," a key pressure point that is on the breast bone just below the nipples and is often touched. The immune system and the thymus gland are stimulated by strong, circular massage of this area, which also warms and expands the heart. When a man's chest region is stimulated by affectionate contact or his awareness, it makes him more thoughtful and aware as he makes love and makes his heart feel noticed as well. A guy may allow his heart to be pierced by love when his chest and breasts come together and can visualize receiving energy from the lady via his heart.

Breathing and kissing

When approaching your partner during foreplay, it is very pleasurable to deliberately breathe slowly and deeply. You may get in touch with your body and your partner by taking breaths in and out of your mouth. Breathe deeply into your hands when you touch someone or as you are being touched. Feel the awareness of the breath permeating the cells as it wraps around and penetrates the hands. Try new breathing techniques since they will help you to awaken your life force and urge you to be present in your body.

A crucial component of foreplay and romantic creation, kissing is a genuinely delightful and sensuous art. It may even take on a life of its own. Profoundly, it arouses the desire for sexual activity. The closest you can go to being face-to-face and eye-to-eye is via kissing or being linked at the lips. As it is such a private act, people often hesitate about kissing someone after having their heart broken. We seem to value kissing more than sex, almost as if it were holy. There is often an intense desire to kiss each other during a romantic act if we are in love. The bodies link in an intimate circular completeness via the deep energy exchange that occurs when one drinks with pleasure in the mouth.

Then again, we go beyond kissing like we do when making love. Kissing is most helpful when one feels at ease. Ensure that your lips are relaxed, enabling them to be soft and responsive. Furthermore, remember to relax your jaw and mouth. Typically, while kissing, one person purses their lips into a tight rosebud, and the other person rapidly kisses them on their constricted lips. When the lips are too stiff, this isn't truly a kiss; it's more like a physical exchange of energy via the mouth. The lips should be loose and malleable, yielding and receptive. Bring the lips together very gently while kissing; allow them to meld together softly, with flexibility, and meltingly. They may respond to each other in a luscious dance if they maintain this juicy touch.

The famed French kiss, which involves kissing each other on the tongue, is now highly valued. On certain times when the sex energy is flowing intensely, this is kept in Tantra, nevertheless. An aggressive tongue pushed into a woman's lips at the start of a kiss might be unsettling. She needs to take it gradually; it's too much, too soon. Even more so in the case of a male, kissing with the tongue has the power to immediately arouse desire. If you want to keep the sexual temperature cool during foreplay and lovemaking, you need to be aware of this. Men often utilize the protruding tongue in place of the penis, particularly when it's difficult to enter the female and when he believes their penis is insufficient.

Leaving the tongue out of a kiss may first seem awkward or incomplete, but soon you will be able to sense the excitement and sensuality of the juicy lips themselves. You will be astounded at the consequences on your own body and your partner's reaction if you penetrate your lips with your presence and awareness. Be playful, naive, and naïve while approaching love. Be young and inexperienced. Share a bed, kiss, hug, and even a nose-to-nose massage!

Separating in consciousness

It is crucial to understand that parting slowly and with respect is just as significant and necessary as getting together slowly and with respect. Both before and after play are the same thing. Conscious lovemaking generates a highly powerful energy field surrounding a couple, and if that energy field is abruptly disturbed, it may be incredibly upsetting and have the exact opposite impact. Deep bonding, nurturing, and healing are produced by personal interaction. For instance, it may be physically and psychologically shocking when a man abruptly removes his penis from the vagina, leaving the woman feeling disconnected or suddenly abandoned by her partner. The advantages of lovemaking can also be readily erased. Keeping in mind that the energy fields are one, prevent abrupt separation. When you want to physically detach from your spouse, let them know, and move gently and deliberately.

Following sexual union, lying down next to each other in awareness and relaxing in quiet is very good. Before dispersing the energy through speech or laughter, keep your attention within and concentrate on the body's stream of sensations. This has altering effects and substantially enhances your sensitivity and awareness.

KEY POINTS

- A woman's body warms up slowly and appreciates loving foreplay.
- Keep the sexual temperature cool; it's not what we do, but how we do it.
- A slow, conscious approach expands the body energies.
- Include the positive poles, especially the breasts.
- Breathing, kissing, and touching awaken the senses.

CHAPTER SEVENTEEN

PLEASING AND PERFORMANCE

WE ALL QUESTION WHETHER WE ARE GOOD LOVERS. We question ourselves, "Do I please my partner?" We want to be appreciated and liked, which puts pressure on us in bed. "And am I good enough or am I too much?" We want to do it properly and successfully. Yet, the focus on the outcome and final product has also led to performance and pleasing because of the importance that has been put on them. We are not in touch with our core, the source of the sex energy, when we try to design an outcome based on a concept of what should happen. Instead of heating up and growing inside of each of us, the energy is directed or leaks outside in performance.

The demand to perform rests mostly on the guy because of our physical disparities. He has a heavy weight to bear since he must always maintain a full erection for intercourse to occur. Men's extreme suffering is palpable when they talk of sleepless nights during which they tried everything to get an erection. Men often experience nervousness, which is not unexpected given that we cannot make love or enter without this amazing happening, which further develops the idea of performance.

This mentality implies that a guy must be a good machine to be a good lover. It demands that the male put on a good performance, put on a nice show, and give the woman a good ride. As a consequence, the guy starts to focus on "doing," or making things happen, and as a result, he becomes mechanical. His need for the outward extension of his penis causes him to focus his energy outward since he feels he must get as hard as possible as fast as possible. By doing this, he loses his awareness of his body and his capacity to unwind and have faith in it. It is thought that for love to exist, a man must take some kind of action. But, we must make a fundamental change by bringing the focus back to ourselves to accept a new approach to making love. One of the most fundamental miscommunications between lovers is the penis' focus on its difficulty for love. In actuality, the penis will readily get erect or, at the very least, hard enough for penetration when it is in loving, comfortable sexual conditions. Furthermore, keep in mind the lovely prospect of mild penetration in situations when none is required. The statement "When my penis is soft, I don't even believe it to be a penis" made by a guy in one of my groups is untrue. The penis always has energy, regardless of how hard or soft it is.

Forget the performance, be in the awareness

For a guy, sex has increasingly become a mental experience. Since he has been so preoccupied with evaluating his performance or engaging in fantasies to arouse it, he has seldom had the time to feel his penis. He's been near it and used it, but he's not been there. With this new perspective, where performance is no longer necessary, he can now focus his concentration on feeling the wonder between his legs. He may begin to believe that he is really, and not only in his mind, his penis within the vagina.

It has nothing to do with performance and nothing to do with size, but when he combines his awareness with his penis, it becomes very sensitive and observant. Sensitivity is a plus rather than size when the genitals are regarded as a single entity and as generative organs. As they adopted a new method of making love, men claimed that many of the typical sentiments of competitiveness between them and the display of their physical ability vanished.

Since a woman does not need an erection, she is not required to perform in the same manner as a male. While dryness is readily overcome, she is aware that she must get moist. The performance demand on women is much lower since lubricant or saliva will do. She will start performing for him, however, since she knows that she cannot have her guy without an erection. She is well known for fabricating her orgasms. Since she believes she is turning her guy on and is expecting he will remain harder for a longer period, she may also pretend via noises and actions that she is loving the way her man is stroking her or thrusting into her even when she is not.

Most women have done this; some have even experienced actual pain during sexual activity, but they choose to ignore it. Rather than being aware of what is occurring in their bodies, they continue to be preoccupied with satisfying the guy to support his performance. My vagina feels relaxed. What if I didn't go ahead and backward? Consider allowing him deeper access. How can I adjust the angle of my pelvis? As a woman becomes aware of herself during sex, she will realize that many of her motions are directed toward the male and titillating his penis rather than toward herself and her receptivity in her vagina. According to Tantra, a woman's penis will naturally get erect when her vagina is relaxed.

There is a greater chance of attraction and reaction in environments that are flexible and permeable.

There can never really be a sexual energy exchange between two opposing poles when a woman's energy swings away from herself in pleasing and a man's energy is thrown forth in performance. Rather than the long, gradual, sensuous burn that Tantra envisions, both are off-center and away from home and are more likely to experience an explosive fast boom.

We're all aware that too much air and wood will cause a fire to burn too rapidly. In addition, we are aware that it won't burn at all without air or wood. For a fire to burn brightly into the early hours, the ideal ratio of wood to air is required. If we think about how making love works, we can see how much love and understanding is required to maintain constant awareness of the wood and flow of air.

We've been taught that the best way to go forward is via excitement. This "hot" energizes us before penetration. Much more heat is required to keep the erection going after the penis is within. We start a fire quickly and stoke it as much as we can to make it burn even hotter. But more importantly, we are igniting a false fire when we produce heat in another person's body before producing it in our own.

Experience your body from within

The bond to your own body will take on a great deal of significance as you gradually remove projections, forget about them, and return to yourself. You may focus on unwinding, breathing, and getting to know your body more deeply. You are igniting your fire when you focus on your own problems instead of the other person, over whom you have little control anyhow.

Before attending to someone else's fire, you must take care of your own needs. You'll then get a huge surprise! Reach out to your partner while your fire is ablaze. Continue starting your fire as you get closer; if they've started theirs, there may be blazing golden embers. You'll get really helpful answers if you keep asking yourself, "Am I doing this for myself, or some concept I have about me?" Drop back into your core whenever you catch yourself projecting outward, pleasing, or acting, and you'll likely both feel a surge of sexual energy go through you.

The time for penetration is usually a sensitive one, and here is the place where the demands of pleasing and performing may readily show. When the bodies and energies are ready for penetration, the minds are often consumed with worries regarding penetration. Is the timing right? Is it likely to occur? Does it work? Does she mind if I enter? It happens often that a guy may touch his girlfriend before she is physically or mentally ready, which can make her feel pushed and make her resentful of making love. It's crucial that a woman be open to being entered to lessen these constraints and raise knowledge. Couples should bring their lover inside as soon as the lady is ready, I advise. If the male is upright, great; if not, more time is required, and the lady may wait.

Alternatively, you can agree to attempt mild penetration. The guy is more likely to be ready because of his active, positive love polarity, while the woman is often more passive sexually and requires more time than her partner. As the woman makes a move toward penetration, she enters as a receptive and willing partner. It must be noted, however, that the woman must not refuse her man's penetration as a part of a push-and-pull power struggle. In the Tantric philosophy of love, this will introduce the aspect of the mind and its desire to dominate the other. The act of making love should be done really and honestly by partners who are trying to build a fresh foundation for their relationship.

The hint that a woman suggests penetration is incredibly good for both men and women. Guys appreciate it because it puts the burden of duty on the woman, allowing them to unwind and not worry about finding the right opportunity to approach her. It's valued by women as well. Now that she is free from the need to use excitement to prepare herself, she can relax. There is no chance of crossing limits since it is obvious that admittance is up to her. A guy will notice the difference when a lady accepts him inside her vagina, and the wait will be worthwhile.

As heightened sensitivity develops and the expectations to perform and satisfy decrease, you'll discover that the penis and vagina quickly adapt to this new strategy. Lay next to each other for a while, let your eyes contact, take a few breaths, and then unwind. At this point, you are both prepared. It seems as if the organs comprehend that love is now being given to them. Their natural reaction to one another is triggered when they realize they are now the ones who must fulfill the demands of love. Normally, mental stress prevents this instinctive reaction. Very subtle events eventually become more than sufficient to arouse sexual energy without requiring the other to satisfy or put on a show for you.

Pleasing and appearances

We live in a culture that is fatally obsessed with physical attractiveness, and women in particular feel intense pressure to fit in with its strict expectations. Once again, this results in an objective and external perception of who we are, and we become disconnected from our inner world, our subjectivity, and the source of our beauty. Physical characteristics are just a small part of true dazzling beauty. That is an inside quality that shines. When a lady is deeply in love, she is radiant with affection and extraordinarily attractive. It radiates despite the appearance. A woman's physique embodies the graceful, empowering contours of femininity.

The seeds of true beauty, elegance, and dignity are planted by awareness and a loving attitude toward one's own body. But the majority of us criticize or compare our bodies rather than loving them. Forget about the usual and begin to appreciate your body from the inside out while admiring others' shapes and features. Relaxation and acceptance have a significant impact on the body's energy, which produces distinctive feminine beauty.

KEY POINTS:

ᘓ Forget about being a perfect lover—without a goal there is nothing to prove.

ᘓ Redirect that same energy into feeling your own body from within.

ᘓ When a man and a woman are relaxed and receptive, loving is easy.

ᘓ The radiance of love is the true source of beauty in a woman.

CHAPTER EIGHTEEN

ORGASM AND EJACULATION

In the Tantric setting, the topic of an organism is significant and prone to vehement debate. There is considerable doubt that the main motivations for making love in traditional sex are ejaculation and climax. Both of their pleasant feelings are calming and assist to release tensions. They also aid in restful sleep. When you take them away, it seems as if there is no reward and that the enjoyment is being taken away. Sex without ejaculation is unthinkable for many men and some women.

But, intercourse is ended when a male ejaculates. The chance to be near and to exchange energy has just vanished. Why come here and regularly discard your semen, the Tantra asks at this very point, "Why to finish it here?" Keep it inside of yourself because it is your life force power and pure energy. You don't need to assist the body in ejaculating; it will do it on its own if it needs to.

After ejaculation, many men claim to feel exhausted. Our culture makes jokes about guys falling and snoring once they arrive, but the reality is sad but genuine. Yet, we strive to put a stop to the sex act. There is no denying that because of our training, our lovemaking has the propensity to be goal-oriented. We are motivated by the need to relieve internal tension as a result of restless excitation. We experience sex as if nothing occurred if we don't have an orgasm or an ejaculation. That wasn't a true or fulfilling sexual experience. As a result of feeling tricked and subject to your lover's whims and demands, you can become unsatisfied, irritated, or argumentative, particularly if your partner arrived when you did not.

Since they allow us to relieve internal stresses, orgasms, and ejaculation become addictive. While it feels fantastic, have you ever considered your true feelings around the desire for an orgasm, beyond the obvious pleasure? Do you have to be here? Even if I don't show up, do you feel as if you have already made love? Being associated with or linked to the approaching experience makes it challenging to progress in the tantric method since you have a set destination in mind. Tantra's guiding principles state that there is nothing to do and nowhere to go. This orientation allows for the easiest emergence of the Tantric experience.

A peak experience—a circle of desire and release

The pinnacle sensations are orgasm and ejaculation. They result from a planned accumulation of sexual energy leading to a release, which occurs consistently in the same manner. The overwhelming need or want for orgasm causes us to be spurred onward by the mere concept of it, which inhibits creative or passionate lovemaking. And with deliberate effort, we climb the ladder of excitement, where every bodily cell and thought is directed toward achieving ever-greater heights.

Friction is utilized to develop and increase the genital feelings, which are the only subject of attention. When sexual tension swallows the body, overflows over, and releases in relief, this is challenging and determined labor toward a transient paradise. The reason why the sexual experience remains limited and empty and makes it impossible to feel greater pleasure and joy is because of this unconscious drive for a climax. We are ignorant of how severely our sexual indoctrination has conditioned us, which is why this powerful orgasmic need feels to us to be so natural.

The wisdom of our genuine sexual nature, which is based on ingrained polarity, is suppressed by conditioning (mind), which has given rise to the craving for the climax. When your body prepares to have an orgasm, pay attention to the tension and constriction it experiences. Observe how your tummy and pelvic floor are constricting, as well as how your buttocks are becoming more constricted.

Yet often after returning, you and your partner feel even more distant from one another, as if you had been abruptly parted. Darkness now hovers over you in place of the enticing sparkles that were formerly in the air. We may question ourselves, "What was it all about?" In reality, many partners experience dissatisfaction and sadness when they consider coming but ultimately decide to leave. We keep coming back empty-handed and without something, which fuels greater yearning. We often lack the luxury of actual sexual connection and instead find ourselves in an unending cycle of want and gratification.

Most of the time, a woman is unable to reach a satisfying climax quickly. She moves more slowly than a male because she has full-body sexuality that encompasses her breasts and is dispersed across her whole body. She won't be able to have an orgasm spontaneously unless she can engage in a sexual dance while making love. Time and rest are necessary. Insecurities about their non-orgasmic plague many women throughout their whole lives. Women are plagued with the orgasmic phantom. Several women have pretended to have orgasms when they haven't even experienced one, much less many. Articles addressing the challenges of orgasm are common in women's magazines.

The main issue is that while making love, women get much too tense, which is exacerbated by the effort of attempting to get closer and by concentrating on the clitoris. It's not a sensation to be pushed or sought to experience the blissful orgasmic waves that reverberate throughout the body or the increased vaginal sensitivity that develops as we melt into the breasts, where we nearly bottom out.

Presentness is necessary. It is a release of sexual tension, not the sensation of pleasure that may be experienced via vaginal contact with the penis, that results from an orgasm that is reached by generating excitement through friction and stimulating the clitoris. Although some people are better than others at becoming tight and at de-escalating that tension, an orgasm is not truly an orgasm—it only seems that way to us!

It is misunderstood that older women have less desire to push or force a sexual release since it seldom makes sense to make the effort. Women are immensely happy to learn that they don't have to orgasm and that they should even forget about orgasm. As a result, they can now fully unwind and resume their sex lives. Several claims that they instinctively understood that orgasm could not account for all of the circumstances. Women may also gain by ignoring the clitoris and allowing it to engage as and when it is triggered by the organic touch of the bodies. When we stop thinking about orgasm as a goal, we may more easily connect with our fundamental orgasmic nature.

As they often ejaculate too quickly, whether it is within fifteen, twenty, or twenty-five minutes, males tend to have the opposite issue more frequently. However, it is still premature to ejaculate before penetration, whether it occurs five seconds or thirty minutes afterwards. For a guy to have true sexual fulfillment or for a woman to access and activate her magnificent sexual energies, there just isn't enough time. The fact is that orgasm and ejaculation may occur or not since the bodies are built to make love for several hours without any kind of goal or purpose. Not out of habit, but by your decision.

Relax and stay in the now

Tantra encourages us to temper our enthusiasm and let go of the results, recognizing that sex is about more than just fleeting pleasure. No doubt about it. You may not have any experience with it yet, but when we let ourselves relax into sexual energy, we offer ourselves the option of keeping the energy within the body. To try to get rid of the mechanical nature of orgasm and ejaculation, ask yourself the following questions: "Where am I now? Am I focused on this moment or the next? Am I able to feel this stroke, this penetration, or am I thinking about the next, and the next, and the next?" The answer will come to you in an instant!

When making love, ask yourself these questions often and observe how your focus is split between your climax and your partner's enjoyment. Recognize that being in the present moment right now is different from being somewhat ahead of yourself; understanding this distinction is crucial. Regain awareness by bringing your attention back to your center and inside. To meet your partner, you must now project this awareness outward from a place of inner stillness.

It is often questioned why a woman shouldn't travel if she doesn't lose her semen, which gives life. That will be OK if she is totally at ease.

Understanding the connection between couples during sexual activity is necessary else. It's challenging for a male to remain uninterested in ejaculation when a woman is focused on generating orgasm via excitement. Inside the genitals, there is a fundamental conflict of interest here. The man's relaxation will be overpowered by the woman's degree of excitement (tension), and all of a sudden he becomes ecstatic and prepared to ejaculate. Penis tension increases as the vaginal environment does. Even if a guy can unwind during his partner's climax, she can end up being less engaged and excited than she was before. The fire has abruptly died down due to a dissipation and energy leak. A woman is absent and not present or responsive when she is concentrated on having an orgasm, which is more significant.

Unsurprisingly, relaxing is the key to Tantra. If you relaxed into the valley and transformed into an ocean wave instead of aiming for the summit, what may happen? The source of your sex energy is reached when you let your body relax, which also causes a lot more to occur, such as starting to move away from your polarities.

Sexual release is biological, so there's nothing wrong with it. Yet, when we let it take us along or overwhelm us, we lose sight of the journey of love that comes along with it. We stop thinking about prolonging the ride because we are so focused on the summit. It's the difference between tearing through the forest in a sports vehicle that misses everything except its velocity and taking a leisurely, unhurried, and satisfied stroll through it while taking in the sights, sounds, tastes, and sensations that you encounter. We lose ourselves in the journey and let the destination find itself when we focus on the little stages that add up to the total. If so, each time is unique.

Choose a new way to make love

Tantra provides us with the chance to play with life energy. It is not about setting limitations and telling you what not to do. The message is, "You've done it the other way so many times; how about trying something different for a few months? If you don't like it, nothing is lost. In the meanwhile, let's play a bit and see what happens. Maybe the ancient lovers who embodied and communicated Tantra understood something you didn't."

Tantra provides you the option to choose a different method of making love because it recognizes that frequent ejaculation calls for a man to act outside of his masculine polarity. As a consequence of his constant efforts to raise his sex energy to its highest level and the imbalance that this causes inside, he loses some of his masculinity. He is often left weak and unloving as a result of this. Some men embrace this, believing that the weariness and feeling of isolation that comes after sex are the norms, while others despise it and use it as motivation to discover their untapped potential. If a guy can use his brain to guide his sexual expression, he opens up a nurturing universe for himself and his partner that goes well beyond achieving goals and killing time. Men have claimed to me that when ejaculation frequency is decreased, they experience a rise in sexual desire and a matching increase in vigor. Not in the opposite direction, however. He has a newfound sense of vitality, confidence, and loving manliness, and his desire does not go away as it usually does; rather, it intensifies and deepens.

Whilst the terms "orgasm" and "ejaculation" are sometimes used interchangeably to describe the sensation for males, a man's ejaculation is not an orgasm. Semen alone contains the physical component of orgasm; the mental and spiritual aspects are entirely ignored. The opportunity for sex is greatest in this area. In an orgasmic experience, the body is no longer seen as a physical substance; rather, it vibrates like electricity-like energy that is luminous. You are a limitless, pulsing, dancing force that is absorbed by the divine.

The body turns into steam, vibrating in time with the lover, the hearts pounding in unison, and suddenly climax occurs—two become one—a circle vibrating in unison. This is the traditional representation of yin and yang, with yin sliding into yang and yang into yin. In our habitual need for orgasm, we are unintentionally seeking precisely this spiritual condition because, during the few moments of orgasm that we experience, we have the opportunity to submit to a higher power.

An inner ecstatic phenomenon

Tantra provides an orgasm that is a state rather than an experience. Rather than experiencing an orgasm, it is more concerned with becoming orgasmic. One lasts forever, the other for just a little moment. An inner experience called ecstasy is the source of immense happiness and contentment. It is a valley orgasmic experience, a sinking into the euphoric depths of calm. And maybe from this, a peak might emerge from the depths, forging and whirling its way up orgasmically to its apogee. An orgasm without ejaculation is possible for men in this valley of calm. While the semen is still within the body, the orgasmic energy travels through it in waves and has no physical component. At times of pleasure, ladies are known to discharge a lot of liquid, heavenly nectar known as "amrita". That is the beauty of a valley orgasm: one cannot purposefully seek one. It is a by-product of the intensity of being and deep relaxation, not something that is done. You are not the cause of what occurs to you. With the help of the Love Keys, we may actively take efforts to decompress during sex and open the door for such a potential encounter. And the easiest way to go about it is to not always choose orgasm or ejaculation. Rest easy, be mindful, and observe what transpires. That does not imply that you will never return.

It implies that you prolong your romantic relationship and reserve your ejaculations for much later, or that you come less often, possibly gradually. As you get more engaged and involved in a variety of stimulating and gratifying activities, including lovemaking, your interest in or dependency on the peak declines. You must keep in mind that when we suppress the sex energy, we are essentially empowering ourselves.

An important and motivating step is being able to recognize the precise instant an orgasmic or ejaculatory urge begins. You may truly start to play with your sexual energy if you can pinpoint the precise instant when excitement suddenly sweeps over you and fills you, almost like a substance to be felt in the body and luring you further. You have a choice in how to make love when you understand this particular point. Going with the urge and fostering it would be the obvious course of action. If you want to do this, make sure you do it fully awake all the way through.

The less apparent option is to unwind, although this is challenging. The struggle with biology and conditioning results in a greater liberation. Relax as soon as you sense a craving! And do not wait even a moment. If the need is supported for even 30 seconds, the want is driven toward release, and it is challenging to reestablish the present since passion continues invading.

Instead, to fully profit from this potent Tantra instruction, you should confront your desire as soon as you become aware of it and immediately give it up. Release all tension throughout your body, including your jaw, shoulders, tummy, and feet. Every part of the body is relaxed. Men may reroute their energy by concentrating their consciousness on their third eye or solar plexus, respectively. The more you relax inside, the less pressure the sex energy is under, and as a result, it inverts and rises inside of you seconds later, a moving force that fills you with energy. The greater the thrust, the deeper the relaxation. An exciting energy develops out of excitement. The art of Tantra is to ride and unwind with this power. It becomes motivational, meditative, and a cause for residing and loving. Hence, the sexual energy starts to deviate from its predetermined route if you can start to enter with awareness, capture the instant when the body begins to execute its program, and then relax deeply. You are about to have a magnificent surprise when it starts to valley out and spread. Continue to unwind, and you'll discover that relaxation is the most thrilling activity available.

It's good to explore the Love Keys when you do ejaculate. The awareness has an impact on the experience's quality. This acknowledgment puts the process into direct focus; tell your partner, "I'm coming now." Examine her eyes. Transmission of energy via the eyes. Be sure to share it with others. Relax the muscles in the buttocks and the ones at the base of the penis, move more slowly, or even attempt to stay motionless. The experience will grow if you do this.

Following that, stay laying next to each other, hugging, with your penis in your vagina.

Maintain your focus on your genitalia and let them exchange energy when you're sleeping. As a male approaches, a woman will often make more effort to have an orgasm at the same moment, although this seldom succeeds and always falls short by a few strokes. To properly receive masculine energy into her, the woman should unwind and be loving. The sensation alters for the male as well if her vagina is supple and responsive. His penis will feel more vibrant and active with enlarged feelings in a calm, undemanding atmosphere.

Discover the joy of going nowhere

Making love while resisting our impulses becomes easier with practice. The more "present" you can be, the more magical the lovemaking will be, you'll notice. After some time, being "here" starts to seem more normal, and the thought of traveling seems like a big effort. When you reach a certain point, it seems as if you slip under your training and the overt aspects of sex to enter a more tranquil but alive state. It gets simpler to let the bodies make love without the mind dictating a certain course. Also, you maintain your ability to have a typical orgasm and ejaculation when you are stimulated. If you'd like, you may turn it on at any moment. Excitation reaches its pinnacle as a consequence, and the body expresses this as well. Other possibilities and choices exist, but we won't be able to see them until we learn to relax into our sexual energy and allow it a chance to act independently. The sexual energy is no longer crushed outward in release, but starts to pivot, impressing itself inward and upward until our sex center returns to its innocent and natural form, at which point it has been cleansed and "deconditioned." One gets the impression that the sex center is no longer being constrained or held down by anything. Once liberated, sexual energy is unrestricted and has no bounds.

The degree of presence and available sexual energy determine the manner the bodies pick. There are moments when everything is calm and tranquil, then the next instant enormous movement emerges from the center of this stillness. Each movement—a stroke, a shove, a penetration—was given total relaxation in and of itself. Going nowhere while being ferocious and furious.

A wonderful celebration of the body that fully embraces the present moment is what true passion is. To be wild while being mindful of it is to say that wildness is wonderful. Real wildness is only here, here, and here; it has no purpose or direction. When bodies escape time and enter orgasmic oneness via presence, divisions vanish.

KEY POINTS:

- There's more to sex than orgasm and ejaculation.

- A man's ejaculation of semen is not true orgasm.

- A woman's orgasmic potential expands with receptivity not tension.

- The energy of desire can be inverted to thrilling effect.

- Forget about orgasm and become orgasmic through relaxation.

CHAPTER NINETEEN

NON-EJACULATION

Ejaculation being seen as a way to unwind is one of the things that confuses people. Yet in reality, it is a dissipation, a massive loss of energy that causes exhaustion or irritability instead of the revitalizing quality characteristic of rest. The non-ejaculatory phenomena, the retention of semen in the body, and reabsorbing the life energy into longevity were all recognized by ancient Taoist teachings, according to which a man achieves good health by living in harmony with the world. The non-ejaculation, which is distinct from ejaculation control, is also of importance to Tantra. In the case of non-ejaculation, ejaculation is not often a topic of conversation. Due to the way you are letting things go, it is not a problem. Because of this, romantic relationships may last a long time and be very fulfilling. Contrarily, regulating your ejaculation suggests that you have a powerful want to ejaculate that has to be repressed. After the sex energy has been purposefully increased to its height, stopping the ejaculation becomes an act of pure will in which mind control is used to overcome the sex energy. It is distressing, to put it mildly, when a woman finds herself at the whim of her partner after hearing him yell, "Stop! Don't move!" All she wanted was for that one more stroke to occur.

The notion of continually managing ejaculation, of dancing on the edge, and of toying with fire is the basis of many practices that go by the erroneous label of Tantra that is being practiced today. Nevertheless, males report experiencing congestion and aches and pains in their testicles or groin, which is not a very desirable outcome. The energy is turned on and off, on and off, as the whole system is prepared for release, and this is why it occurs. Although this "dance with danger" might make you feel good and energized right away, there often follows a comparable low. A clogged-up residue of tension in the vaginal and abdominal region persists, and as a method of lovemaking, it ultimately may exert stress on the prostate gland, resulting in pain and medical issues.

Controlling one's ejaculation cannot be a soothing experience since the term "control" itself indicates stress. The stress of the urgent ejaculation and the tension of trying to control it mentally result in a double tension. The pleasures of Tantric lovemaking come from letting go of the sex energy and entering a condition of acceptance in which nothing is forced. It emphasizes a slow, smooth growth of sexual energy via sensuality and relaxation; excitation and tension are not part of this vision.

The positive and negative polarities of the genitals confront each other via their intellect, resulting in a state of natural euphoria during sex. Below the ecstasy, the sex organs start to work. Other than that, nothing is promised or fixed in advance. Although some days have a timeless or drifting aspect, other days it is electrifying or completely engrossing in intensity. Ejaculation feels astronomically distant in this kind of sensation.

Orgasm and the ego Regrettably, it has become socially acceptable for both men and women to see their partner's orgasm as a result of their creative efforts. Also, a male thinks that a woman's orgasms reinforce his sexual ego by demonstrating that he is a better man. Yet when he insisted that she come to please himself, he restricted his sexual potential and kept a woman circling the surface layer of her sexual energy. The door to major change is still shut.

Nonetheless, even if they are unable to ejaculate themselves, women still like seeing their male ejaculate. Many claims to feel tricked and as if the male is withholding something from them if he does not ejaculate. Or, more often, they utilize it to complete the sex act since every woman is skilled in inducing her partner's ejaculation. This mentality reveals the woman's desire to dominate her male and to persuade him to stop producing the life-sustaining semen that gives him the ability to exercise power.

She has been conditioned to attempt to govern things while being unaware of her divine feminine power. The woman finally gets the chance she's been waiting for to start making love with feminine receptivity and within her polarity, as the guy becomes less connected with ejaculation and as it becomes less significant to him. She naturally exudes calm and elegance, and she learns about a new sexual realm that is far more enjoyable than searching for an orgasm. Her euphoric and luminous state of authenticity makes her the wellspring of love. Her life and her partner's life might both be altered by this.

The desire to ejaculate will undoubtedly come and go while you are having a romantic relationship, but a desire is not the same as an intense drive. The body's need is a need, while desire is still only a notion in one's head. Please allow ejaculation to occur if you find yourself in a liminal space where you are unable to unwind while in a romantic relationship due to a strong or recurring desire. Expel your ejaculate while being conscious. Feel every minute and enjoy it.

Tantra says it's better to ejaculate since resisting it will just result in twice the stress when a guy is battling with himself and attempting to control his impulses. This tension will probably reappear the following time, leading to a cycle of tension, such as uneasiness after sexual contact. If the male has to ejaculate, it is preferable to simply do it since tantra promotes relaxation of the body and mind. He will then soon have the opportunity to restart.

Intense, pure pleasure, particularly during deep, prolonged penetration, is likely to sometimes be felt by a guy when he learns a new way of perceiving his penis. The intensity of the feeling is so overpowering that it nearly makes him feel excited, and he may feel tempted to go with it and go for it while the vaginal walls are being awakened with love and awareness. Nevertheless, men have discovered that if they truly feel the penis, behind this surface of excitement the sensations are of a radically different character, the source of enormous delight when the male positive energy begins to go into the woman for the first time. As a result, it is often well worth it to maintain your composure and refrain from ejaculating when the desire arises.

How do you feel afterward?

Be led by how you feel in the moments and hours after an orgasm or ejaculation as you start to play with them. I started experimenting with orgasm and my lover's ejaculation, sometimes going all out and other times not, and I started noticing how I felt afterward—not immediately after, but even much later. This was helpful knowledge, and I learned that when I did not force an orgasm, even when nothing seemed to have occurred, I felt better. As a general rule, asking yourself

"How do you feel when you do?" and "How do you feel when you don't?" is beneficial for males as well. You'll find all the solutions in your experience. It serves as your primary instructor.

KEY POINTS:

- As a man relaxes, the powerful urge for ejaculation decreases gradually.
- Non-ejaculation is not to be confused with ejaculation control.
- The first implies relaxation, and the other tension.
- Controlling the urge for ejaculation suppresses the energy with possible congesting effects.
- Non-ejaculation increases vitality and creativity.

CHAPTER TWENTY

PREMATURE EJACULATION

Typically, PREMATURE EJACULATION is characterized as ejaculation that occurs before mutual pleasure. This might be as basic as ejaculating right after after penetration or suddenly and uncontrollably ejaculating. The precise duration varies for each person and might be 10, fifteen, or even twenty minutes. Whether or whether the act is complete, it finishes. In a manner, there isn't enough time for sexual development. Although though premature ejaculation is a very normal occurrence, many men experience horrible solitude while going through it. Men need to understand that the issue is primarily psychological in nature.

The issues here are not with the body itself; rather, they are with the repressions of sex, the tensions around it, and the lack of knowledge. A guy experiences significant presexual excitation as a result of these tensions and fears that impact his thinking. The male ejaculates uncontrollably when the opportunity finally arises because of the intense internal pressures, worries, and concerns as well as the overpowering sexual arousal.

Think for a minute about the fundamental idea of polarity to get an idea of when and how this occurs. The male's positive energy leaves the penis and is absorbed by the female into the negative pole of the vagina. A disturbance has developed in the woman's vagina, making it expecting and demanding since she has been depending on movement and clitoral stimulation for her sexual experience. Not to mention the tensions from our shared history that are submerged in unconsciousness.

In foreplay, when we add titillation and excitement, the disruption manifests as tightness and tension in the vaginal walls, which arouses a need or hunger of sorts. Occasionally this may grow to the point where it really hurts, and the whole region seems like it is contracting and becoming smaller. As a result, when penetration happens, the woman is not just full of energy and nearly protective, the circuit for the passage of energy is broken.

Understanding sexual arousal The guy joins the woman's disturbed vaginal environment with his own social tensions and enthusiasm, and he is now excessively positive. He encounters an unusually agitated or aroused charge here. Male energy no longer has a place to go and cannot flow into the vagina. As it encounters opposition on its way to where it needs to go, it prematurely bursts into ejaculation.

Understanding the woman's potential role in causing early ejaculation, whether unintentionally or knowingly, is crucial. Any time during the course of the sexual encounter, a sexual image or intense stimulation can cause this excitable charge to move in the woman, causing the energy to rush down in a wave of excitement and leading to the man's sudden and unexpected ejaculation, almost as if it were being pulled from him. Conversely, a woman has the capacity to consciously increase the sexual tension in her vagina at any moment, forcing sex to be had. When this sort of conduct cuts the possible link to her femininity, there are consequences, of course.

The condition of the woman's vagina informs the penis immediately on how to act when the guy enters her. The male will get agitated and tense, which will increase his likelihood of coming if the vagina is stimulated and tight and protective. The penis reacts to this invitation with an exhilarating life energy, with positive flowing into negative, if it is calm and relaxed, smooth and accepting. One cannot overstate how crucial it is to comprehend sexual excitement. You will be freed from its unconscious hold once you start to have the ability to recognize it as and when it emerges. Instead, you may use it to your advantage and provide clarity and knowledge where there has previously been compulsion or confusion.

Simple rules should be followed in order to prevent premature ejaculation. Prior to making love, men and women shouldn't become too excited. It's also suggested to begin with mild penetration. Fear and tension are both decreased when two individuals do away with the internal demands and expectations of sex. Making a date to have a sexual encounter also helps since it lessens the man's worry about the potential for having a sexual encounter. Knowing that he doesn't need to convince the lady causes him to feel less nervous or hesitant. Excessive excitation and the occurrence of premature ejaculation are directly related to the tensions, anxieties, and concerns of this kind. When there is no temptation or persuasion, we may engage into lovemaking knowingly and with more ease, and with time, our bothersome habits from the past start to fade away.

If there is no worry, the act of making love might gradually endure for hours.

You both need to maintain as much relaxation as possible while concentrating on basic contact, sensuality, and touch, as indicated during a recent look at foreplay. Instead of stimulating the breasts and genitalia, touch them in a manner that respects them and kindly says hello. In this calm condition, sexual desire will naturally and wonderfully arise. Awaken rather than excite. Penetrate as soon as there is a sexual reaction. She should know you are erect. If she's prepared, ask the lady. Tell the guy you want him inside you right away when you're ready to do so.

Instead of each individual making their own assumptions, it is really helpful to work together in this manner. It is preferable to infiltrate well before you both get really eager. Ejaculation is less probable due to the absence of enthusiasm, which keeps the genitals cold. Avoid spending too much time in the first phases of making love by penetrating as soon as it is acceptable.

In order to maintain your presence, make the first penetration as gradual as you can while maintaining eye contact. It is advisable that men concentrate their focus on and in their penises and not worry about where they are inserting them. His thoughts about the vagina are immediately filled with all of his sex-related connections and desires, which once again trigger ejaculation.

With one lady, some men realize that they ejaculate relatively quickly, while with another, they may go for extended periods of time without ejaculating. Many guys will have questioned why this is perplexing. The lady herself, and not the male, is usually to blame most of the time. It greatly relies on the surroundings in which the penis is situated. The vagina is tranquil, warm, and quiet when a woman is at ease and uninterested in excitement or climax, and intimacy may last for hours. Premature ejaculation is extremely probable in women who have a tendency toward excitability.

As you can see, women greatly influence a male's propensity to ejaculate too soon, thus it's in your best interest to avoid getting your boyfriend too worked up. Man becomes a stronger lover at that point, and a woman is content to the hilt. If we attempt relaxing into the sexual energy rather than stimulating it, we will benefit from it so much more. Regrettably, she has learned via training that love is all about clitoris movement and stimulation, being agitated and energetic, and searching for an orgasm. She believes that the male is also seeking for this. She doesn't seem to think of relaxing into the more receptive, feminine side of sexual experience as enjoyable. The gateway to bliss, however, starts to slowly open up when we learn to remain calm during sexual activity and help the male do the same.

Allowing the guy inside your vagina as soon as feasible will help to prevent anticipation from growing and will increase the likelihood of a longer-lasting sexual union. Invite penetration when you're ready for it both physically and psychologically. Communicate. Invite him to pierce you. Allow for a very gradual first penetration, and after he is within, keep your muscles relaxed while picturing your uterus as soft and receptive. Make no unnecessary movements. Be less extroverted and more physically present, responsive rather than demonstrative.

This does not imply being passive or laid back. Instead, allow your body and what is occurring inside of it—the whole beautiful phenomena of it—be your focus. It will surprise you that this internal glimpse is worth far more than the results of frequent pelvic motions. Your bodies become relaxed and pleasurable as soon as your awareness enters the environment. Take your time, don't rush, don't attempt to stir up the energy, and don't push anything. Just turn on sufficiently, enter and be penetrated, and then maintain this initial desire by being in the present, putting your body first, and use any of the Love

KEY POINTS:

- The cause of premature ejaculation lies in sexual tension and anxiety.
- Reduce sexual anticipation and excitement prior to penetration.
- A woman unknowingly contributes to premature ejaculation.
- Introducing a conscious relaxed approach can eliminate this problem.

CHAPTER TWENTY ONE

ERECTION AND IMPOTENCE

Some men struggle to get an erection, while others do not. Some can obtain an erection merely by thinking about it, while others take a few tries to get one. Some men find it simple to get an erection with one lady but difficult with another. It may be a perplexing, misunderstood phenomenon that both men and women experience as a cause of great suffering.

The worst aspect of this misunderstanding is that most men—though certainly not all—assess their manliness concerning their ability to be erect and pleasure a lady.

Women often have the same opinion about males. How intensely and for how long can he push himself? For a male, all of this functions as a tremendous weight; it consumes him and causes him to question his ability to love a woman, to the point that he even starts to doubt her. The authenticity and naturalness of his sexual expression start to be compromised by his mentality. He slowly begins to feel an enormous amount of strain and stress, but unfortunately, the fact is that a woman is also in charge of a man's erection.

The power of sexual magnetism without excitement

Our perception of sex could change if we start to see the penis and vagina as a single organ, opposite halves of a single entity with magnetic intelligence. It would be more appropriate for a guy to think of his penis as a tool for love that reacts to the love in his counterpart, the vagina, rather than a mental pressure steadily building up in the man that demands he must do something to make love.

This implies he trusts love and waits for an erection to swell and expand either within or outside the vagina rather than forcing one by acting in a certain way. Erection is incredibly effortless and requires no effort at all when the vagina is filled with awareness and love. Amazingly quickly, the penis searches for the recesses of the vagina. Women are aware of how to be attractive or provocative to assist a male to become hard, and they voluntarily engage in these behaviors to facilitate sex.

Nonetheless, her efforts will generally be ineffective if she keeps her attention on the male rather than herself. Women sometimes ignore an essential truth when they attempt to induce an erection in a guy using their hands or mouths, for example. Her vagina, this vital organ inside a woman, determines whether or not she gets an erection; man is simply one component of this wondrous occurrence. What will work is the enveloping velveteen silkiness and welcome liquid feel of the vaginal cavity.

It is feasible to tell the difference between an excited and a powerful erection, according to males who have engaged in both excitement-based and relaxation-based lovemaking. In contrast to the second, which they claim feels brittle, rigid, and yet simple to lose, the first is elastic, flexible, and sensitive. That is comparable to the contrast between a snake's vibrancy and a stick's lifelessness. A man who had been experimenting with the Love Keys once made the astute observation, "I get two different kinds of erections. The first way, is I move into relaxation and non-doing, and after a while, a movement of energy happens and an erection is there. This kind of erection does not go soft when there is no movement. The other way, I move into excitement and tension, and I get an erection that feels hollow because it is not connected with

Another man in one of my workshops said, "When I consciously push an erection by tightening the perineum and the anal area, the energy becomes concentrated in my pelvis, but when I remain relaxed and conscious of my entire pelvic area, the energy falls back naturally and the perineum does its own thing. It still feels the same, which at first was confusing, but when I let it happen, it is like I am available to it, rather than forcing it. I can feel a contraction.

Experience an electrical surge of inspiration

The penis fitting so well within the vagina, for example, allows the energy to flow freely and the erection is a byproduct of the attraction. This is due to the design of the sex organs. Not only inside the vagina but also close by, an erection is possible. The penis naturally prods and thrusts forward as it enters the vaginal area. This is a positive energy seeking its complementary counterpart to feel whole. Men have referred to this polarization of the penis, where it reacts via polarity, as a trip from the head of the penis to the root of the penis. As a result, the magnetic phenomena spreads across the whole penis. When a man can see his penis as a shaft of awareness or a stream of light emanating from the base of his body, he begins to become more cognizant of its whole length and feels alive throughout it.

The penis reacts to changes in the environment quite quickly. The vagina's presence and relaxation can be felt, as well as when it is absent. It can tell when a woman is attempting to have an orgasm, for instance, when the vagina is shifting out of polarity. The guy will often suffer an abrupt loss of erection as the open, loose surroundings of the vagina become tight and restricted from a receptive attitude to a demanding one. The sensitivity of a conscious penis cannot accommodate such a demand and will become less responsive as the erection weakens. Even fully erected, he may even flop out to the side in a moment of unexpected indifference.

The minute the woman's awareness leaves her vagina, the male will often start to lose his erection if the penis is laying erect within her. It is that sensitive in the penis. One single idea may be to blame for this loss of erection. I've been astonished several times by how the penis will rapidly contract the moment I let my focus wander. That makes sense since its electrical twin has vanished or absented itself. The penis will extend out and gently slither up into the vagina once again, recovering lost ground when I can stop thinking and re-engage with my body.

Both men and women are capable of sensing this phenomenon, which causes the penis to be extremely sensitive to the energy in the breasts. The penis reacts right away when the breasts are stimulated. This is due to the vagina becoming open and sensitive as the breasts become more vibrant and positive. As a result, the man's energy may be transferred from the penis into the vagina.

The lady will notice that the penis responds quickly with more energy as the electricity goes within while she is concentrating on her breasts and accepting the male. The penis will feel a surge of energy, a fire, or inspiration as a result of this intensification of polarity, even if it lasts only a brief period. When a woman's breasts are fully open and loving from the inside out, she will feel as if she is piercing a man with love via her breasts, chest, and heart, triggering his heart and love in return.

This demonstrates how the health of the vagina affects the health of the penis and how much more ecstasy both men and women will feel the more present and conscious they are during the act of making love. Making love can be a sign that you are not present if it seems a little dead. Maybe you're worn out or distracted, but you're not loving your partner. The more comfortable you get with entering "here," the more alive your genitals will feel to one another.

Psychology and impotence

Man's biggest fear is impotence. A guy is surprised when his penis cannot or will not function properly, when no amount of stimulation or excitement can make it happen, and when time films, skimpy apparel, or seductive equipment will also not work. A guy who was formerly thought of as a stud might often be shocked by this. Yet here is where impotence will most likely manifest itself. The problem is that the penis has lost its sensitivity and responsiveness as a result of an overreliance on excitement, and if a guy hasn't fully explored his sexuality from the inside, impotence is likely to take hold. Sadly, he has developed an immunity to his sexual energy; self-doubt begins to set in; and frustration and rage escalate. Nowadays, millions of men experience impotence, a condition that is just as common as early ejaculation.

Impotence is commonly attributed to the lover, the comfort of years spent together, the routine of old habits, the layers of emotional walls, and the suffering of silent heart scars. The original love that brought two individuals together all those years ago is now unavailable, and there is a decrease in stimulation and attraction. Also, we now think that older men who leave their marriages for younger women need to be revitalized. Yet, the cause of impotence is not the partner; rather, it is a psychological issue and a result of the penis' lack of sensitivity.

When sex just doesn't work anymore

Tantra informs us that in the event of impotence, the penis is no longer acting as an actual positive masculine pole; it has become flaccid and unresponsive and lost its intrinsic curiosity and sensitivity. It no longer has a foundation in the boundless reservoir of sexual energy. The genital organs are now insensitive and numb as a result of years of sexual misinterpretation and abuse. Men have never been taught how the penis functions within the vagina or how to cultivate the natural magnetic qualities that would offer them and their lovers enduring love and fulfillment. Sensation has long since replaced sensitivity.

A guy who lacks erectile function has no other alternatives; his enjoyment is now limited to sporadic, shallow, and transient moments of release. His sexual dreams and imagination, which are mostly responsible for his being erect, have diminished. His sense of feeling is not what is occurring, but rather what he thinks is happening to him.

Saying that sex just no longer works in today's society is acceptable. Sex is brushed aside as if it were inconsequential, but the absence of a willing, expressive sexual energy quickly develops into a source of self-doubt and is the root of conflicts and emotional unhappiness in relationships. When a guy doesn't engage in sexual activity, he will soon experience the negative consequences of his stagnated energy and develop restlessness, boredom, critical thinking, an easy disposition, and a quick temper.

A crucial aspect of males is left unexplored and undernourished when they make up for this by devoting all of their sexual energy to work and success, leaving little time for love. Later, although surrounded by worldly prosperity, they reflect on their dissatisfaction and issues with impotence, obesity, and drunkenness. They suddenly realize that their priorities are out of order, despite how vital they had felt the money was.

Overcoming lack of feeling together

Tantra holds that male impotence is caused by both men and women. Both male and female genitalia have become more hypersensitive as a result of years of friction-focused lovemaking, and their muscular tissues have tightened and hardened. No tingling, vibrating, sensitivity or mild awareness will exist while the penis is immobile in the vagina. Friction is necessary for the penis to grow erect after years of rough contact because, without it, there are no emotions, no sensitive sensations, and no natural energy. The polarity effect, which disrupts the bio-energy, deadens and makes the erection response unavailable. Thankfully, impotence is a condition that couples can work with together. It calls for self-respect, empathy, and patience. Respect your body, your energies, and your genitalia, and allow them time to recover and find their equilibrium. Set a date to have sex often. Give each other plenty of time and alternate massaging your penis, testicles, and breasts. Be mindful and unhurried while you unwind together.

Lay in bed and attempt penetration without getting erections when you're both ready (described in chapter 12 on Soft Penetration). Once implanted correctly, even the head is sufficient to retain awareness in the penis and vagina and to engage in energy exchange via eye contact. A guy must heighten a woman's consciousness by stroking her breasts to remind her to keep awareness in those areas as well. Repeatedly using this method of seduction will result in an erection that responds to the vagina from this neutral location. It will offer you a motivating understanding of the beautiful occurrence of erection and the solution to impotence, even if only for a little period initially.

It may take many tries before the positive and negative start to react and behave as intended, so stop expecting instant pleasure or results. But, the inherent wisdom of the sex organs may be restored when a guy can start to unwind in the atmosphere of love with his spouse and learn to trust his penis. An erection will once again happen naturally.

Unfortunately, science has developed an incredible "impotence medication"

—a guy needs the typical sexual stimuli or provocation before getting a full erection, hence it is not an aphrodisiac! In the short term, this does provide solace, but when you consider that male polarity is what gives men their ability to erect themselves, the obvious fact is that medical intervention just makes things worse and provides no understanding of the energy truths at play. The guy, who has a history of being insensitive and oblivious of himself, is now transformed into an erection machine, furthering his lack of awareness of himself and, obviously, his partner. The dullness in the penis prevents the activation of her euphoric sexual energies, even though she could be pleased to receive penetration once again. It also doesn't inspire affection.

Insensitivity resulting from tension and anxiety

Men sometimes tell me they have a "sexual ailment" that causes them to have strong erections but almost little sexual sensation. This implies that an erection may last for extended periods, but since the penis is so insensitive, it is unable to develop enough sensation to cause an ejaculation. Thus they continue to pump despite the lack of a few genuine pleasure-filled seconds, which makes them furious. Even if it seems contrary, in a way this might also be categorized as impotence. A guy is essentially impotent when he has a steel-hard erection but there is no awareness present in it. He feels less macho in situations when he does not see his male pole reacting to a lady. A buddy of mine who had severe emotional suffering as a result of his insensitivity from his formative sexual years was lucky enough to encounter a lady who was open to experimenting with him 20 years later. After eight months of making love without the stress and worry that had caused his insensitivity, he was happy to see that his penis was starting to recover its natural sensitivity, able to perceive the environment around it, and react appropriately.

He started to see his penis as a conduit for heavenly energy that could sustain love and profoundly awaken the lady inside. Even the smallest change in awareness (which relieves the burden of our sexual training) is repaid with the vigor of fresh life and sensitivity because the innate intelligence existing in the body is a force so strongly integrating. The body is inherently eager to reclaim its original biological oneness.

❧ Erection is not a mechanical function but a polarity response to the woman.

❧ The woman influences erection through consciousness in the vagina and breasts.

❧ Erection is the natural outcome in the presence of consciousness and love.

❧ Impotence reflects the man's extreme insensitivity to himself and to his partner.

❧ Soft penetration is very helpful in restoring a man's trust and sensitivity in his penis.

CHAPTER TWENTY TWO

FEELINGS AND EMOTIONS

A journey from the mind to the body and from thinking to experiencing is what TANTRA IS. We shall become conscious of the existence of two different categories as we immerse ourselves in the realm of sensation. There are emotions like grief or annoyance that have a strong emotional component, and there are sentiments that are just the body's energy moving about. The Love Keys can help couples identify both types of emotions as they use them. They will see a matching rise in body sensitivity and awareness as they progressively expand their consciousness in the act of making love.

This results in a wide variety of new interior sensations and experiences, including smoothness, velvet silkiness, heat and warmth, excitement, tingling, bubbling, lightness, fluffiness, coolness, molten gold, streaming brilliancy, and the erasure of all physical boundaries. When our demand for pleasure in sex decreases, we become more aware of our intrinsic sensitivity and begin to sense a universe of unexplored feelings that are hidden within. Once the energy starts to flow through inside circuits, this causes sexual pleasure. At first, couples do not define their sexual encounters as being purely sexual since they change completely. One of my workshop participants recently exclaimed, "That is incredibly touching, and it is not like anything you see in the movies," after having his first taste of it.

Our feelings are different from our emotions

Emotional feelings are a very another affair, and they often confound people since they might appear to produce paradise and hell. Love and conflict keep becoming entwined, and it seems like there is no way out of the quiet days. Our emotions and sentiments keep upsetting the peace. This component of who we are, this delicate and often unconscious layer, has to be made conscious. The first two phases include being aware of the body and the mind. In comparison to the third stage, knowledge of our complicated emotions, temperament swings, and changeable moods, this one is very simple.

Even though the terms "emotion" and "feeling" are sometimes used interchangeably, this is a mistake. The distinction between experiencing an emotion and experiencing a sensation is significant. Understanding this difference is crucial, especially in the context of romantic relationships, since it sheds light on our psyche and may help us begin to accept full responsibility for our actions. You can know what is occurring and when it is happening if you know the difference. Emotions are an unconscious manifestation of the past, of something that has already occurred, while feelings are a representation of what is occurring right now, consciously in the present. Emotions function on an unconscious level, while feelings are aware. When emotions are expressed, it is frequently overpowering, disruptive, or unpleasant because feelings are conveyed quickly and innocently whereas emotions are suppressed or delayed in their presentation.

It is obvious that feelings and emotions have very different qualities, and give us almost opposing experiences of reality. Through our feelings we expand our energy, we feel light and energized. We feel connected to others. While emotions like to place blame and say "you always... it is your fault... while feelings take responsibility and say "I feel" or "I need.

How ignored feelings become emotional monsters

Our sentiments, in whatever form they may take, are almost completely ignored by ourselves and others in our culture, which prioritizes reason and reasoning. Regrettably, most of the time we work to suppress them to hide our flaws and limitations. Early in life, as we learn to keep ourselves together, we start to deny our genuine emotions. This is particularly true for males, who are thought to exclusively belong to women's territory when it comes to emotions. The English saying "maintaining a stiff upper lip" is no laughing matter since the upper lip and chin will shake shamefully when we are in touch with our emotions, our fears, and our shortcomings.

When emotions like pleasure, love, or even despair or annoyance go unspoken, they steadily build up and form a storehouse of emotions that interfere with the balance of the mind and body. No matter how much we try to suppress them, it is difficult to ignore these prior feelings in the body. Jealousy, anger, hate, fear, and wrath start piling up early in our lives (often connected to sexual interference). We have become rigid, brittle, and defensive due to the absence of honest speech in society. Our bodies are distorted and our psyches are damaged as a result of the sorrow and disappointment that would make us cry and howl being stored inside of us as emotions and burrowed into the unconscious.

These suppressed emotions remain within us and eventually resurface as negative sentiments. The simplicity of the present is always tainted by the ghosts of the past.

This explains how a person who first seems calm and sensible may explode at the smallest provocation, erupting impulsively into a wave of violent anger. They are letting go of the pressure of old emotions that they can no longer control, and the severity of such an outburst is seldom in proportion to the trigger. If we can become aware of the impact of our past on our present moment we can start to distinguish between emotions and real feelings. The accumulation of stored and unexpressed feelings is released with the force of this pressure behind it, making the person act completely "unreasonably," but in reality, they are acting "unconsciously."

Expressing our feelings as we experience them

On the other hand, emotions are deliberately articulated at the moment they are genuinely there. It is neither hidden nor suppressed but rather made public. A few seconds of a healthy scream from the belly may be very freeing if there is any anger or fury present. There is no residual bitterness that continues to nag at you after the fury has gone. On the other hand, you feel elated and full of life which makes your heart race. An animal-like shriek of agony can help make the situation more palatable when it is an aching, shattering heart. The pressure inside is released. Sincere tears are the expression of sadness. We are liberated from any negative repercussions when we express our deepest emotions exactly as we are experiencing them inside of us. Even unspoken love or pleasure quickly becomes depressed or sad.

The idea is that although our unconscious emotions contain our hell, our conscious emotions contain our paradise. We construct our hell by holding back on expressing our heaven. Although feeling accepts suffering and utilizes it to heal, emotion acts as a defense against it. Heaven may sometimes seem to be hell in the shape of a tragedy, a loss, or a calamity, but if we let the true emotions surface—the agony, grief, and anguish—we feel much better, even inspired. Otherwise, when our emotions go unspoken, they consume our hearts and bring down our spirits. Unless a memory is triggered by an event, these emotions continue to exist as unconscious feelings. The best we can hope for is to learn to express our emotions and therefore get away from them.

Storing feelings in the body

These sentiments go unspoken within the body, which serves as an innocent "home." Internal pressure is produced as a result, and the tension it causes may have a serious impact on one's physical makeup and the range of motion of their muscles. Body tissues are where emotions are stored when they are not expressed. The internal emotional strain affects a person's posture, including the angle at which their jaw is set, and how they carry their heads, shoulders, and pelvis. The gait, the angle of the pelvis, the form of the legs, and the alignment through the knees all show signs of the sexual center being bent due to emotional strain, which occurs in all of us. Yet, a large portion of our repressed emotions is held in the solar plexus, which weakens our energy and physical structures.

The uncomfortable gnawing feeling of being uneasy, as well as a never-ending twisting and turning, may be felt when we are emotionally aware and attentive to the solar plexus. Before, it was claimed that a Love Key for romantic intimacy would be awareness and relaxation of the solar plexus since this would heighten the intensity of the sexual energy and presence.

The solar plexus may also serve as a gauge for emotions in everyday life. Great insight is provided. If you notice a physical sensation, such as a tugging or hooking in the solar plexus, you may be sure that something is up and that the sense of calm has been disrupted. You've got feelings! It doesn't have to be a spectacular incident, and the solar plexus never misinterprets the circumstances. A neighbor making fun of your kids or pets, a friend ignoring you in a coffee shop, or a spouse who is too busy to kiss you goodbye might all be examples of mild examples. Later on, you could realize that you're feeling uneasy with a sense of loneliness or dissatisfaction, particularly in your stomach.

Awareness, acceptance, and relief of tension

Instead of lugging this pain about with you all day, name the exact emotion you are experiencing—abandonment or insecurity—and allow yourself to experience it, including the bodily side of it. With mindfulness, go towards the solar plexus and immerse yourself in the sensation there. Imagine flames in the base of your belly burning it up as you stay with it for a time. Check-in with yourself later to assess how you are feeling. How do you feel about yourself? You probably felt some comfort and a sense of lightness of spirit after bringing awareness to the source of your feeling and acknowledging it.

You are once again anchored in your being when the bodily weight dissolves and the tension is released by accepting it. There is nothing left to do in this situation, so you may go about your day with a happy heart.

Yet, you may need to phone your spouse and let him know you miss him, or you might need to talk to a friend to find out how they're doing and to express your emotions. You could also find out that they were so preoccupied with their morning woes that they failed to see you at the coffee shop. The whole situation abruptly vanishes in a cloud of smoke. What was offending was your sense of insecurity and desire to be respected and recognized.

And this sparked the feelings that had been there all along. You may need to take further steps to get rid of the pain if you discover that just admitting the sensation is insufficient. Always engage in some physical activity for a few minutes, such as hopping about, stomping your feet, punching a pillow with your fists, or even babbling to yourself incoherently. The undermining influence of emotions on the body is greatly diminished by any motion and sound.

With a bit more acute awareness, we may begin to think about our feelings, our moods, and our brief ups and downs. As emotions are a layer in the body, this calls for great attentiveness and is challenging. We feel that they are an essential part of who we are and that they define who we are. It is crucial to maintain awareness of the solar plexus to release any associated tensions in the area. Awareness is also very helpful in identifying subtle emotions. Otherwise, they build up and harm our minds.

The act of expressing emotions is always advantageous since it relieves the body of internal stress. Nevertheless, the ties connecting us to our unconscious characteristics start to fall apart when we become aware of the feeling rather than the emotion itself. This observation reveals the progressive demotivation of emotions. The past continues to exist. When emotions originate in the present, they are thus free from the impurities of unfinished previous experiences and may be expressed in their original, unadulterated form. As a result, life and love start to seem innocent and simple.

Love, emotion, and sexual healing

When we start a sexual act, we do it under the stress of all our repressed emotions and our now-fragile internal emotions. Our emotions are unintentionally aroused and put into action when we engage in sexual activity, casting shadows over our lives that we are unaware of. As a consequence, we continuously engage in the same disagreement or feeling of discontent with our partner, feeling as if we are going in circles. Perhaps, since the same problem keeps coming up, you will be cut off from several partners you have loved and abandoned. We can't seem to do it correctly.

Yet since we don't understand what love truly is, we've come to believe that its ups and downs are a necessary component. We may start to take greater responsibility for our love and separate it from the emotional region when we become aware of the repercussions, especially the origins of our emotions in the past. By bringing knowledge and understanding to the act of love and letting go of our identification with our emotions, we may begin to build it from scratch.

The genitals of both sexes are weighed down with guilt and accumulated negative emotions that conflict with the natural polarity, even though it manifests differently in men and women. The genital poles will begin to relax after we relieve the strain on the penis and vagina by eliminating the compelling urge to engage in sex. The emotions that have been bottled up will start to emerge in various ways as they do this. A guy should not be ashamed to weep or express his emotions, and he must be as truthful and straightforward as possible. Your lover will appreciate you revealing your vulnerability, particularly because you'll likely notice that your penis is more sensitive and aware while you're crying.

As a young man going through puberty, a male buddy of mine observed some markings appearing on his penis. He was so distraught that he believed something was wrong with him. There was no one he could discuss it with. Moreover, he was unable to know if the marks were completely normal since he had never seen a penis other than his own. He needed to visit a doctor, but doing so would require talking to his parents first, which was impossible. It was only when he started to make love intentionally that this humiliation and anguish started to emerge from his body.

Instead of burying his shame and mortification, he continued to feel his penis as being "sick" well into his late thirties. When it did, he understood how these feelings had impacted every one of his intercourse with women. The vaginal tissue may mend on its own when you allow yourself to experience what you were unable to feel years before. A new sensitivity develops in the genital organs as a result of the flood of tears that serve to wash away the pain and rid the body of internal pressures and pollutants.

When the poles gradually clear out, they restore their original polarity by removing their disruptions (negative awareness). In this manner, the lady gets more feminine while the guy becomes more macho.

How the past can disturb the present
The discovery that a significant number of women had experienced sexual abuse—many times as very young girls—in

my work with individuals has been quite upsetting. Yet to a lesser extent, males too experience this unexpectedly often. Many people carry into adulthood the suffering and perplexity of traumatic early sexual experiences. They often struggled to communicate their sentiments of terror and panic to others or to share them with others. The next-door neighbor, the uncle, the brother, the father, the grandpa, or even the local priest may have been involved. As an alternative to trusting a complaint of sexual molestation, mothers have been known to accuse their daughters of being sexually provocative. These potent impressions, which underlie all subsequent interactions, are imprinted in the body and mind. Years after the occurrences, suppressed emotions have evolved into sentiments that might come to the surface and demand release to be free of the dark, clandestine past.

The foundation of sexual healing is the emergence and release of old emotions, wrath, anguish, and disappointments, the remains of which have left an impression on the sex organs. The relaxation that we seek may and will bring up unpleasant memories to release the tensions that are preventing an otherwise unhindered flow of energy. With this knowledge, we can accept the buried trauma from our childhood and the old wounds that are beginning to show themselves as the genitals start to repair themselves.

Achingly deep tears flowed from my eyes as I felt my suffering, and there were moments when I contorted violently and uncontrollably, trembling, shivering, and sweating. Even if I still don't know the exact events that caused the pain, I discovered that it was more important for it to be released than it was to be the cause. Healing occurred as a result of letting go of long-repressed emotions; my vagina experienced a melting sensation and tenderness.

I've always said that discussing things in bed is inappropriate since this is a love story, not a therapy session. The best course of action for me was to continue making love as the tears were streaming, keeping myself open to the penis bringing up these memories from my past. My tears would stop flowing if I turned away, crumbled into a heap, or attempted to speak about it. I would then feel hollow or unfinished. If I remained in the moment while making love, confronting my partner and the intensity of my feelings, breathing deeply, and letting the vulnerability and tears, I would be able to reach a deeper layer of suppressed feelings. My vagina began to feel and perceive more as the layers came off, and my partner's penis also started to react.

Noticing emotion as it arises

It's critical to notice when the unconscious and the past enter the picture and when emotion is at your door. It all depends on how you respond to it. For instance, an old feeling could be aroused when you are making love if your partner touches you hard or without consideration. This might bring to mind an uncaring uncle who did the same thing to you when you were a little girl. Even the slightest movement might reveal anything. You may have sensations of disgust, curiosity, dread, guilt, fascination, or agony when you suddenly encounter the uncertainty and trepidation of your childhood experience. The ugly scarred foot of the past has stepped into the beauty of your current love, and all of a sudden, without surprise, the two of you are on completely different planets. Completely distinct. It almost seems as if you have entered another personality and that communication is almost impossible. You scarcely even know yourself, much less your partner. He used to be here, directly in front of you, but now you can't look him in the eyes, as if you're staring through a long tube. You may get a sudden sense of being in a fighting mood and blaming your spouse for your misery due to an overflow of unspoken emotions.

This is a clear indication that feelings from the past have intervened and momentarily disrupted your current experience. Even though you can feel awful, the fact is that going through these feelings can be helpful since the process is eventually uplifting. I advise you to attempt to reach the true sensation that the emotion is concealing or shielding as soon as you realize (and this becomes simpler and easier) what is occurring. If you experience fear, you could discover that deep down you feel completely abandoned and alone; if you experience anger, you might discover profound despair. Let this long-buried emotion come to the surface and take possession.

If you can't go back to it right away, admit where you are to both yourself and your spouse, for example, "I'm emotional right now, I'm feeling apart," but don't participate in any kind of blame or presume that you made a mistake. It's useful to speak about it if it makes the issue better. It is better to spend some time by yourself if the feeling of separation does not go away.

What are you feeling?

When someone becomes emotional, it doesn't take long for the other person to follow suit and explode in anger, both of them blaming the other for all of their failures. This is one disturbing element of emotionality. There has been a steady decline in the situation. A dispute arises unintentionally when one person's emotionality resonates and vibrates with the other's hidden emotion. They each accuse the other of being to blame for their suppressed feelings now bursting out from every pore! When neither party is aware nor clear, communication might become completely impossible. It is advised that you avoid speaking when you are feeling very upset since doing so rarely resolves the situation and often causes further uncertainty and distance. You shouldn't continue talking until you're ready to acknowledge and disclose your weakness. In any other case, it would be far more polite to recognize what is taking on and to take a short physical break. It may just take an hour for you to complete your stroll.

The previous emotions may need to be worked out over a longer period, such as a whole evening or a few days. You may need to let out your emotions by having a good cry or by beating a pillow to vent your fury and frustration. When you're feeling emotional, it's necessary to move your body. Jogging, dancing, or physical activity of any kind will do.

Give yourself enough time if you need it; don't be frightened to do so. Your feelings of loneliness, abandonment, rejection, and betrayal may become more apparent during these times of solitude if you start to realize that this specific partner is seldom solely to blame for how you are feeling. You have probably experienced similar emotions previously if you are honest with yourself. The situation has altered, but there is nothing new. You could even observe that it is a pattern that develops as your closeness increases.

When your heart yearns to open but is prevented from doing so by the agony of having loved and not receiving the love in return at another time, you go through that agonizing experience that makes you retreat. Your partner isn't directly to blame for what you're going through; we are all living out the past in the present. Your love won't be tarnished by the disappointments of the past when you accept full responsibility for your feelings. When you give yourself enough time to separate, you may walk into the present and have a silent reunion.

These emotions may be relieved as actual feelings and let go of via moving through the solar plexus, the solar ganglia, and the heart. A thick foreign material that swirls and spirals painfully inside, moving through the fascial system, which weaves a connecting labyrinth throughout the body, is sometimes how the emotion is felt physically. The desire to identify the source of sorrow is lacking in emotion, which clings to pride and safety. Yet, if you have the guts to see beyond the feeling, you'll enter the realm of what you once felt, which will make your pulse beat, your breathing quicken, and you could even tremble and perspire. Once that happens, your heart will express itself, its softness and fragility. Then and then, the barrier between you and your partner will fall. You will be reunified just as swiftly as the emotion that was causing you to be apart done. The feeling of being in a different world will vanish as your eyes are met with your lover's. The seed of our reunification with our true selves—the love we are—can be found inside these feelings.

Remember you are more than just your emotions

It's crucial to remember that you are not your emotions while you're feeling them so that you don't over-identify with their suffering and misery—even if it may be hell—and that you can get out of it. Also, don't believe anything you say or do. Emotion enjoys having its way, and because this isn't who you are, you must resist being sucked in. Avoid making hasty decisions or possibly hazardous moves. Mind your language. Recognize that you are experiencing an overpowering cloud of (previous) emotion. The potential of both men and women must be understood clearly. Try to establish a mindset of accepting these emotions as you allow the grief and anguish to rise up and out of your body, realizing that you are relieving your heart of its burdens.

You'll feel more alive, nearer to your partner, and more like yourself as a result of this. It will have a revitalizing quality. We learn to comprehend the swings between happy and unhappy periods when we approach romantic relationships with fresh insight. When we can identify suppressed emotions causing a disruption, igniting anger, argumentativeness, and even physical excitation, we may identify them and save a lot of potential difficulties. Understanding that feelings elicit enthusiasm is essential. Because of the drama involved in a battle, sex is very intense and thrilling during that time. Tantra says that you should never make love when you are in a fighting mood.

Many couples use sex as a last-ditch effort to connect and ease the agony of separation. More emotion and consequent unconsciousness in sex are both readily a result of it. Before making love, give your feelings time to subside. A caring and healing atmosphere like the one provided by the present makes it harder to meet and more difficult to be attentive when making love. Being that mending is a process, delicate emotions may suddenly resurface at any time. If you are not on guard, you may find yourself back in the same situation with the same problems.

Take every opportunity for greater expansion

As emotions occur, the mind might join forces with them as it attempts to convince you not to share them to protect you from being seen as vulnerable. I once wanted to say a simple, profound "I love you," but I couldn't bring myself to do so because I was so ecstatically consumed by love. I forced them down my throat. At that instant, my thinking led me to believe that it was too personal and overwhelming. I shouldn't have made my affection, fragility, or dependency known. A short while later, I saw that my body was starting to contract and that my presence had completely crumbled from despair. I sobbed as I felt my sexual arousal and sensitivity progressively wane.

I lay there, constricted and shrunken, drowning in the recollections of all the times in the past when I had failed to convey my love. In that agonizing experience of withholding, I realized how many chances I had passed up that may have led to greater growth in my body, heart, and soul. Now that I've used those priceless gifts, my heart flies on the wings of love.

We shall experience layers of defense, protection, and agony on the path from our personality to our being, all of which serve to keep us apart from our essence. When we go inward into the center, we must encounter and let go of them.

While some individuals acknowledge to being in a constant low-grade emotional state, these fluctuations are not perceptible, the following is a solid reference to the many aspects of emotion and feeling.

• In sensation, you will sense intimacy; in emotion, you will feel alienation.

• Feelings are a conscious manifestation, while emotions are an unconscious one.

• Feelings are experienced in the present; emotions often pertain to the past.

• Emotion projects blame and says, "You constantly...," whereas feeling acknowledges:

• "I sense-heed.."

• Emotion will employ the same phrases or repetitions year after year; emotion is portrayed in a new way.

• Feelings expressed generate strength and life; suppressing emotions has draining consequences.

• Feelings are the heart, but emotions are the ego.

• Feelings that aren't voiced last just a few hours.

KEY POINTS:

- Feelings expand and connect us, while emotions contract and separate us.

- Emotions relate to our unexpressed past, feelings arise consciously in the present.

- Expressing feelings day by day prevents an emotional overload building up.

- Learning to identify "emotion" brings tremendous insight into relationship patterns. Remember, we are not our emotions.

- Old buried emotions are displaced through consciousness in lovemaking, welcome them.

CHAPTER TWENTY THREE

WOMEN, EMOTIONS AND THE HEART

Women are renowned for having uncontrollable emotions. A guy is often driven to despair by the fact that emotions frequently arise even when things appear to be going so nicely. When harmony suddenly descends into sadness or flares up in a conflict for no apparent cause, how can he love and comprehend a woman? It's a nightmare dealing with women's erratic moods, fighting and nagging, questioning and prodding. It seems as if the lady he loves so deeply is sometimes possessed.

Sex is the root cause of these mood swings. Tantra tells us that by insisting on excitation and climax, a man produces the emotional aspects in a woman that he finds most unsettling. A woman is prevented from reaching her full potential as a woman and is held to the lowest degree of sexual expression. She has been a sexual object and a source of male enjoyment for ages.

This makes her angry and depressed. Her untapped divine qualities gradually grow latent and stagnant over time, and she develops emotional instability due to a profound sense of unhappiness, disappointment, and lack of love that permeates every cell in her body. Traditional sex, which is hot, frantic, and centered on self-gratification, stirs up these feelings inside of her, causing sexual arousal and impairing her capacity to be receptive.

Emotional sex and instability

As a result of the residual tension that excitement leaves in her body, she becomes explosive, volatile, and unstable. This explains why couples may easily get into heated disagreements just after sex.

The inability to relate will come as a result of the sexual tension eventually dissipating, much like static electricity. Sexual unhappiness is, in reality, the foundation of the majority of relationship issues.

Although emotional intercourse, as it is frequently referred to, may be highly wonderful, it only lasts a few seconds and eventually drains life energy. It could make you unhappy and give you a sensation of being apart from your partner, making you lose interest in them. We are grieved by it because we know in our hearts that we have exploited one another rather than made love. This increases the emotional weight we carry, making it difficult for us to love others in the present because we are so consumed by the ghosts of the past.

A woman's emotional instability and recurring patterns are so ingrained in her that she starts to think of them as who she is. Her emotional side has grown to be who she is. Women get the misconception that their lives take on shape, structure, and significance when they experience a particular level of emotion. People mistakenly believe that when there is conflict, love is also there. Contrarily, although this belief is also untrue, women often believe that if there is a time of peace and tranquility between them, then the love between them is fading. A persistent theme of dissatisfaction is often the emphasis of a woman to gain attention and breathe new life into the relationship. To get a sense of movement and a feeling of love, she will create a small tug-of-war or push-pull situation.

Women who are emotionally charged during sexual interaction become more excitable, which makes it challenging for both men and women to unwind and enjoy being in love. Once it has finished its phase of spiritual nourishing, orgasm will be a constant call. The corresponding emotionality of a woman gradually decreases when sexual energy is permitted to relax rather than being forced into a peak. She feels content, calm, and fulfilled.

It is during this transition from linear (sex energy released) to circular (sex energy retained) that a woman feels more like a woman—more radiant, loving, and feminine. The true source of female sexual energy and ecstasy is located in this circular movement, the union of sex and heart. Unfortunately, women rarely fulfill their feminine potential because neither she nor their partner recognizes or makes use of the crucial female polarity in sex—awakening sex energy through the breasts and heart—which awakens sex energy during physical contact. She intuitively understands that romance and sex can lead to a lot of possibilities. She feels a divine union that is blissful and orgasmic, where love reigns, and she longs for this state. Though she continues to be fundamentally dissatisfied, her distress eventually manifests as emotion.

A woman will become more emotional and emotional in personality as excitement and goal-oriented sex continue in her life. She will demand love but never feel the contentment of love. Since we have lost our inherent capacity for love, this is a tragedy on the deepest level. True orgasmic bliss, where a woman feels her body pulsing with love energy and herself as love itself, is never achieved through passionate, male-oriented sex. In addition, it starts to manifest physically, with a band of tension forming over the uterus and ovaries as a result of sexual arousal. Most women are unaware of this, but years of intense sex and forced orgasm cause the ovaries and lower belly area to become extremely tense and crowded.

A woman may experience repeated vaginal infections, irritations, or discharges as a result of this, and it may even have an impact on her urinary system. Additionally, the breasts start to become ill because they are not understood in terms of polarity. Her entire personality is impacted as a result of how her hormones and menstrual cycle are affected. A woman and her partner may experience devastating side effects from these emotions, including days of fatigue and confusion. The instability of ongoing ups and downs and a whirlwind of emotions that come with love then come to symbolize it.

Stepping away from emotional patterns

Love is not an emotion, as the tantric teachings make abundantly apparent. Love is more of a condition of being and a trait that you possess. It is calm and not heated, accepting and not demanding, unwinding and not tense, and happy and not down. It is not a request, an expectation, or a change in one's heart. You are a source of illumination, plenty, and radiance of love. It is most beneficial when a woman learns to identify her emotional states, regardless of how dissatisfied, angry, or jealous she may be at the time.

Only then would she be able to start letting go of this intensity of overpowering feeling and this damaged component of her personality, allowing herself to start building a new reality in which she is the winner rather than the victim? She may admit to her partner that she is having a difficult time being trustworthy or straightforward because of how she is feeling. She may be open and ask for anything she needs, whether it is a tender embrace or some alone time. Her awareness of her emotionality may serve as a continual point of reference that she may use as a signal to see danger and change the situation before becoming enmeshed in it. This demonstrates actual ownership of love. A woman might start to feel her deeper loving nature by taking deliberate steps away from the feeling and, in doing so, breaking unconscious habits based on the past.

A woman will fully blossom in her feminine sexual expression if a guy has the guts to maintain his sexual temperature at a calm burning flame rather than a ravenous inferno. Men and women rediscover love when it is unhurriedly allowed to emerge through polarity. Yet it takes a guy with vision, knowledge, and dedication to love for this to happen. He may then assist in bringing back his lover's physical connection to the heavenly wellspring of her love.

A man can only be completely fulfilled by sex when he can see his partner develop as a result of his collection of her heavenly energies, flower, and radiate this love back to him. He now senses a genuine masculine authority inside himself. Similar to how a woman may take charge of her destiny by asking that a guy make love to her rather than merely engage in sexual activity. By gaining this insight, she stops the further accumulation of crippling emotions and opens the door for love to return.

Sadly, this may be challenging since women need love so intensely that we'll take any attentions that pretend to be acts of affection.

Making love in consciousness

It's wise to be cognizant of the fact that feelings will ebb and flow when we make love in awareness. Instead of holding onto them, let them flow through you. The internal balancing process includes this as a fundamental component. Women naturally experience unpleasant feelings more often because of the greater number of sexual traumas they have as a result of their physical fragility. It is typical for women to experience intense, illogical wrath even after an act of conscious affection, which they may be tempted to direct towards their partner— the same guy they had just fallen in love with—in the previous hour. We must and will release these unconscious parts of ourselves that have been kept there as a result of consciousness entering the body. These feelings are replaced by the quiet that knowledge causes in the body. Do not focus these feelings toward or on your spouse; rather, let them flow freely through your body. It would be better to exclude him from the situation, accept responsibility for your actions, and savor the excitement. Enter a spare room, and use your fists to pummel a large cushion. Get up and move about! Nonetheless, be mindful of your body and take care not to inadvertently harm yourself by being as physically active as you can.

Remember that when awareness is infused into the organs of love throughout the mending that is occurring between the penis and vagina. A man may disclose a woman's fundamentally loving nature by using a contemplative approach to sex to combine sex and heart in her.

Key Points:

- A man is largely responsible for the emotional fluctuations of a woman.

- Emotions have their source in the tensions of the conventional sex act.

- Conscious sex reduces a woman's emotionality, her experience of separation between sex and love.

- Acknowledging emotion is an essential step in restoring balance.

- Through loving a woman a man can reveal a new world of love.

CHAPTER TWENTY FOUR

LIFE CYCLES AND SAFE SEX

EVERYTHING IN NATURE IS BASED ON CYCLES OF REGENERATION AND WITHDRAWAL, WAXING AND WHITENING, LIGHT AND DARK, BIRTH AND DEATH. The spectacular act of birth and a calm dying are inextricably linked by the concept of sex. Birth implies reproductive and fertility cycles, both of which have a significant impact on a woman's life. In fact, without these cycles, we would not be able to honor the beauty of love and life as we do today. Reproduction and fertility cause mayhem in the area of love. The interruption of menstruation or pregnancy occurs just as things in love are getting wonderfully creative.

Avoid unwanted pregnancy

All women and men must use proper caution to avoid unintentionally starting a new cycle of birth and death. Lives are changed by it. Nowadays, we are lucky to have several options for controlling birth, and everyone should properly educate themselves about their options by consulting a specialist. A woman finds it difficult to completely relax into the sexual experience because of the subtle dread she has about her ability to get pregnant. This fear keeps her in a constant state of profound tension. After sterilization, several women have said that this was their most notable liberty and that it made a significant impact. Most people were not consciously aware that they were carrying this strain, yet it was nevertheless a huge release. If a male chooses to be sterilized by getting a vasectomy, a woman will likewise go through the same thing.

The likelihood of becoming pregnant is decreased when ejaculation frequency is decreased. This is not meant to imply that not ejaculating is a viable alternative to contraception since seminal fluids are known to include sperm that may move quickly.

One can't help but question, however, whether man's addiction to ejaculation is to blame for the current population surge. Condoms are often the easiest preventative measure that couples can take. Both new and established relationships should follow this rule.

Safe sex

Condoms are also necessary while having sex with a new partner to practice safe sex and prevent getting AIDS or other STDs. Avoid any genital touch without a condom to guarantee protection since genital bodily fluids cannot be shared. You must depend on your abilities, and you must not entrust this task to someone else. The possible danger and suffering that might result are not worth it. Regardless of whether you are a man or a woman, always be ready to bring up the topic of wearing a condom with your partner. At all times, keep a few with you.

To assuage any worries you may have regarding AIDS, being tested for HIV is always useful. Both parties may get an HIV test if a new acquaintance turns into a long-term relationship. We may start by making love to one person today, which is the apparent solution. When we learn the genuine meaning of love, we grow to appreciate the comfort that closeness brings.

Condoms

Condoms, on the other hand, do provide a barrier in the way of things happening naturally since they enclose rather than allow for penetration, which may cause the entire thing to condense into gloomy rubbery folds. To prevent awkward circumstances, this does imply that lovers and couples need to discuss it beforehand. Such communication is critical, especially when testing out new parameters. When sex is acknowledged and concerns go, tension is reduced and rapport is established.

To make things easier for you, be honest with your spouse about your situation. Request whatever aid you need, then provide it if necessary. Waiting till another time may be preferable if making out is not acceptable at this moment. While using a condom, it's possible to lose your erection. Yet, don't give up hope. Apply the condom on the unerect penis once again after a few minutes have passed. Your penis will certainly rise in response if you keep up the foreplay and sexual awakening with each other, at which point you may go on.

In general, it is best to use a condom just before you start making love, long before you have an erection. A soft or semi-soft penis is suitable for the application of a condom, and either the male or the woman—or both—can perform it. To make the head visible, roll the foreskin back and draw all the skin folds toward the base of the penis. Gently pull the condom all the way down as you roll it on.

At this point, the condom may help your penis slowly erect, and you can go forward as necessary when the appropriate opportunity for penetration arises!

Whether a condom's rubber hinders sensitivity is a common question. Unquestionably, given that the penis and its sensitive surroundings are separated by an unmistakable covering. Men still describe the same remarkable magnetic reaction of the penis within the vagina despite the absence of genuine physical touch, indicating that the penis' inherent sensitivity is unchanged. That the penis is skilled and intelligent is indisputable evidence.

Lubricants

Only "designer-style" lubricants with an aqueous basis or specific pharmaceutical lubricants like KY Jelly should be used with condoms (water). Vegetable oil or petroleum jelly should not be used with condoms since these substances degrade the rubber and reduce protection. (Condoms have a history of rupturing or falling apart for no apparent cause.) Get a lubricant that works for you from the variety available on the market. Long ago, the Chinese Taoists utilized oil because it was thought to lower the bacterial population. Almond oil or any other pure, odorless vegetable or nut oil is OK, but condoms should never be used together. While saliva has the most lovely feel of all, it is not always clean. Saliva is useful for emergencies. Because of this, irritations may develop when saliva is introduced into the vagina and the normal acid-alkali balance is disrupted.

Be sensitive during menstruation

Men and women respond differently to the beginning of the menstrual cycle. No universal guidelines exist. Each pair must take into consideration the demands of the other and make decisions that fit their circumstances. Women often have more sensitivity at this time and may fear being abandoned, whilst males may be more afraid of the blood or the chaos of it all. Nonetheless, be kind to one another, give and exchange energy via physical hugs, or lay still and rest in awareness next to one another. The impact of such events may also be profound.

To assist the menstrual flow and prevent it from being reversed, which may have congestive consequences, it is advised that the woman take a posture on top of the male when she is menstruation. Moreover, during this time, heavy thrusting is not advised. The tensions associated with menstruation pain are known to be released by a typical orgasm, but this is just a temporary solution since the pain is often a mirror of built-up sexual tensions. Thus, keep it calm and relaxed so as not to add to the stresses that are already there. A woman's issues with period pain, as well as all of her premenstrual and menstrual syndromes, are likely to improve in lockstep as she starts to unwind in her love life. She will experience an overall improvement in her attitude on life as well as a more effortless ability to give and receive love.

It's possible to observe that our level of interest or passion changes while we make love. Very intense phases that come and go quickly appear to occur in cycles. Rest constantly follows activity in nature's cycles, which shouldn't give rise to misgiving or hatred. It is nevertheless advised to try it out even when we don't seem to feel like it. Examine what occurs when you combine the bodies. In contrast to the body, which is often more than happy to be present and calm, the mind is frequently not. Keep in mind that you have the option to quit at any moment. Even though I didn't seem to feel like making love, I had so many unexpected encounters. So, making love is often better than coming up with an explanation.

In the days leading up to menstruation, a woman often feels emotional and depressed. Considering how uncertain and insecure she is, life may be terrible for her. Since she feels unlovable within, she often views making love as being impossible in this situation. She will release a lot of her anxiety and fears during the sexual encounter if a guy can help her make love intentionally. Menstruation will no longer be a source of misery, and peace and happiness will rule. Being straightforward with a woman when she is experiencing an emotional crisis during her premenstrual or menstrual cycle is crucial.

To help the lady, he must gently remind her of what is occurring and try to keep from showing his own emotions out of unconscious response. What, for example, do you need at this moment?

Physical touch is always a cure-all for the woman because she is lacking love—the driving force behind all emotion—deep down. "What can I do for you?"

Love is the best treatment there is and it works wonders, so make love if you can. Instead of abandoning or blaming her, help her get through the crisis by being there for her and being kind. The guy who is addicted to sexual ecstasy must take responsibility for a lot. Because of this, a woman may now be so easily unstable and unpredictable. It has destroyed the fundamental attributes of a woman. Now, he has to stop this process from happening. Men and women are advised to be as open and honest as they can be to express their feelings to help heal previous scars.

The lesser-known men's hormone cycles go disregarded whereas the women's hormonal cycles are well-known and extensively addressed. Men do experience the blues, and there is evidence that males are affected by subtle cycles that are deeper than those that afflict women. The state of love is so chaotic that it is not surprising. The most subtle influence on him is caused by his partner's hormonal changes, and he only serves to confirm this since he is unaware of it.

His mind and body are greatly affected when she gets entangled in hormonal knots and he is powerless to free her because he is a male. As opposed to this, his spouse will become more loving and sexually open to him as he becomes more sexually conscious. Without regular ejaculation, the hormonal components triggered by sexual activity will be reabsorbed, resulting in physical energy and a loving heart. This manifestation of his manhood has a strengthening effect. The positive, revitalizing power of sex.

Cycles of ill-health

Cycles of genital illness must be mentioned, even if they may appear unconnected. Several couples who have experimented with lowering sexual tension and excitement have seen a commensurate decline in recurrent genital infections. Chronic genital disturbances including Candida, herpes, cystitis, bladder infections, thrush, and unexplained discharges or irritations may affect both men and women. As mindfulness is included in romantic relationships, couples have noted a noticeable shift in the pattern of these encounters. It seems that irritations of the sexual organs lessen as the genital tissues become polarized, relaxed, and healthier. A friend of mine told me, "My vagina is now totally healthy. Before that, it was a constant battle against herpes and Candida. It is amazing. I feel so happy about this because it was a burden for me, for our sexual life, and the relationship." This friend had been troubled by such occurrences for several years.

A close male buddy of mine also had herpes. He felt as if his lack of availability was endangering his masculinity since it followed him about like a shadow and was a continual source of anxiety. He noticed that his herpes breakouts lessened as he started to make love with more awareness and a more loving, respectful attitude toward himself and his partner. He started to realize that if he gave into his training and made love unconscious, a herpes breakout would soon follow. The recurrent breakouts subsided as he became more adept at remaining awake and aware. When something unexpected occurred, he was always able to link it to an unspoken feeling that he had suppressed.

Women's bladder infections are often caused by intense sex. A site for infection is generated when the friction irritates the urethral opening right below the clitoris. When a couple has been apart for a long and upon reunion makes love with a lot of energetic ardor rather than rejuvenated, relaxed sensitivity, bladder infections commonly result. Men and women both experience strain from friction, which finally affects the vaginal tissues. When the charge cannot leave the energy system, it accumulates and causes bodily annoyances or disruptions.

The constant force of healing is relaxation. Sexual energy is rearranged to allow it to flow via inner blissful channels as the finesse of lovemaking improves and the sexual tensions subside. The mind is profoundly affected by this, and peace between the body and the spirit follows. By expanding into the spiritual generative cycle of sexual energy, we can transcend the biological life cycle of reproduction and realize our full human potential. The use of sex to foster awareness of life beyond the body and life itself is the greatest life cycle of them all.

- ❧ Sexual energy and interest is subject to natural cycles.
- ❧ Explore making love even when you don't "feel like it".
- ❧ Contraception and safe sex must be talked about in advance.
- ❧ Non-ejaculation is not a substitute for contraception or safe sex.
- ❧ Loving sensitivity and communication is required during menstruation.

CHAPTER TWENTY FIVE

ALONE ON YOUR OWN

WE MAY WONDER WHAT TO DO WITH OUR SEXUAL ENERGY NOW IF WE FIND OURSELVES ALONE OR WITHOUT A LOVER. How can I remain vivacious and seductive? How do I make room in my life for love? Tantra serves as a gentle reminder that each man and woman is a whole being inside of themselves. In keeping with the polarity idea, a woman's body is negative in the vagina and positive in the breasts and heart, while a man's body has a positive pole in the penis and a negative pole in the heart. The fact that these opposing poles come together to create a magnetic rod implies that energy may move freely between the positive and negative poles.

Deep orgasms provide delight and bliss that are experienced within the body and are reliant on the sensitivity and awareness of the individual. For instance, this explains why a woman can claim to have had an orgasmic experience while her spouse was dozing off and uninvolved. The flow of internal energy is initiated by the mere fact that the penis is in the vagina. This might put a person in a joyful condition if they are highly aware of themselves. Tantra instructs us that if we have ever had a single orgasmic sex encounter in which the sexual energy travels orgasmically inward and upward, we may utilize this same experience to raise our awareness.

An internal recreation of this, including the conscious movement of consciousness inside the body, allows for repeated recall and reliving of a cellular experience that vibrates. Great change is conceivable via this conscious remembering of the orgasmic sensation and the orgasmic energy pouring inside. It is nice to understand that you may intentionally use your imagination to extend the positive benefits of making love.

You might designate a certain time to lie down and listen to yourself and your inner energy if you are apart from your partner for a long. To help the body's energy flow through, use your imagination. You will soon begin to experience streaming through your body, much as when you are in a loving relationship. It will possess a comparable quality. Moreover, it's a good idea to utilize this method of communication with your partner rather than the telephone, which we often use and find to be woefully insufficient. Instead, set a date or agreement to relax and lay down at the same hour, like nine o'clock at night. Although being physically apart, you are still one in your soul. You just need fifteen to twenty minutes, however, you may attempt longer. The outcomes will wow you with their love and renewal. By engaging in this exercise, you are enhancing the love that exists inside you and is a manifestation of who you are.

Resting in consciousness

This movement of life-giving energy throughout your body is achievable if you're alone yourself and unattached. It is highly advised since it directs consciousness inward to help you concentrate on yourself. You will feel much more loving and satisfied just by doing this, which is huge nutrition in and of itself. All you need to do to include Tantra into your alone time is set aside some quiet space each day to relax. Resting and bringing awareness into the body are the goals. Time slips away when we establish this oneness with the subtle energy throughout the body, and inner satisfaction emerges. Not the space in the bed next to us, but rather we feel full. But, to do this, we must maintain our awareness.

Most of us use our time in bed or during a nap as a chance to check out for a moment and escape the stresses of the day. After this form of sleep, you often awaken feeling a little dazed and worse off since it did not provide you with the refreshment you were looking for. We are all familiar with how it feels to wake up in the morning feeling extremely worn out, almost as if we haven't slept at all. By bringing awareness to the body, these effects may be reversed.

The most enjoyable and helpful thing individuals can do for themselves on a regular, even daily basis is to rest in awareness (see fig. 16). It takes at least twenty minutes. Laying down, closing your eyes, and bringing your awareness to live inside your body is all that is required to perform it. Lay on your back with your head, neck, and spine all straight. This alignment is essential since it greatly enhances your presence.

Put a cushion beneath the knees for support so that they are softened and bent just a little. This significantly improves relaxation and makes it possible for awareness to transcend the limitations of the physical body.

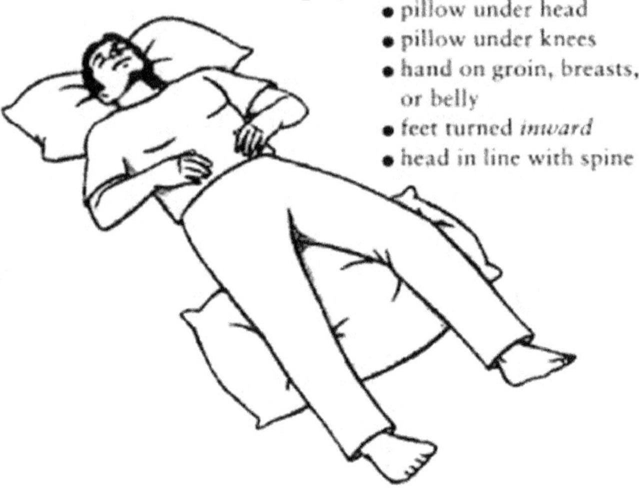

Fig. 16   Resting in consciousness

When you feel at ease, shift your focus from the outside to the inside, putting the day's concerns behind you. Using your awareness, move throughout your whole body, easing and relaxing any tensions you may be experiencing. Exaggerating the stresses by first contracting and tightening the body may be helpful. Tighten and release many times. After sensing the top and lower halves of the body, bring them all together with your mind in the region above the navel. Look within and downward with your inner sight while gradually settling into the physical feelings. It should be distributed uniformly throughout the body.

Maintain your head and neck in alignment. Deepen your breathing, take it gently, and just "be." Only twenty minutes should be spent doing this. You could suddenly disappear into yourself and into timelessness. See how immensely refreshed you feel after such a slumber! That is remarkable. You will notice that the quality of your sleep will be better if you do this before going to bed at night and spend the first twenty minutes resting in awareness. You could sleep less. When you're lying flat, which is a most wonderful posture, even sleeping may become a restorative meditation. With experience, turning inside becomes simpler, and the benefits of resting in awareness make it an excellent live support. As relaxation emerges from awareness, it transforms into a revitalizing and healing energy.

How to connect with your inner opposite pole

Bring your positive pole gently into consciousness and see golden light filling the space to improve this meditation's depth and progress. Men should concentrate on the perineum at the base of the penis, whereas both nipples should be simultaneously focused on women. Whenever you experience a surge of energy or light, you may start to visualize it flowing forth in all directions toward the opposing negative pole. Men could sense it as a series of sudden jumps or leaps of light or energy traveling upward, whereas women might experience it as a slow spreading and rising of energy.

A more euphoric circle of energy forms inside as we do this and connect with our inner opposite pole, our magnetic rod. It could take some time to prepare for this. If you were lucky enough to have at least one prior blissful sexual encounter in which the energy went orgasmically inward, utilize your awareness to trigger this memory in your body's cells. The breath may be added to this positive polarity meditation; a woman can visualize breathing in through her vagina and out through her heart, and a guy can visualize breathing in through his heart and out through his penis.

Ladies in particular should focus their meditations on the positive pole, which are the breasts and nipples. It also starts to rebalance the polarity by bringing forth the feminine energies that are already present in the breasts. The heart center starts to vibrate and expand as the breasts begin to revitalize themselves, surrounding her with a powerful tenderness. But rather than focusing on the heart itself, it is advised that a woman put her consciousness into both of her nipples at once. To open the heart via the breasts has a significant effect on a woman's energy system and ripple effects throughout the body.

Meditating on the breasts may be a very helpful practice for a woman who is alone and misses affection. The inward turning of the consciousness effectively redirects the energy that would otherwise be used to crave love, keeping the feminine energy alive and alert. She starts to sparkle and become more lovely as life would have it. Several ladies have reported having the experience that love found them the instant they gave up looking for it. Love would knock on the door and enter the room as soon as they had come to terms with their circumstances and were being kind toward themselves.

Men and women alike may learn from this that loving oneself is essential. Without first loving ourselves and having the capacity to offer love, which also entails having enough love inside ourselves to share, we cannot expect others to do the same for us.

A sense of compassion and love for oneself is produced when awareness is brought into the body. This makes one more graceful and present.

Exercise, massages, bodywork, and dance are all highly healthful activities that are very helpful in developing bodily sensitivity and awareness when done frequently.

Be receptive to the growing consciousness in your body

Use the Love Keys to aid in the expansion of awareness inside the body. A lot of them, such as eating more slowly, relaxing while brushing our teeth, and strolling, may be employed successfully outside of sexual activity. It is really helpful to keep in mind to relax your pelvic floor when you find yourself alone, to breathe, and to let your gaze alternate between the inner and outside. Several of the Love Keys may be implemented into your life by using mindfulness, and this relaxation will bring about a qualitative difference in your everyday routine.

You could discover that your efforts provide greater results. Try standing with equal weight on both feet and your knees slightly bent while doing something like cleaning the dishes. The warm, wet, soapy suds are surprisingly a sensuous thrill, establishing a bodily presence and anchoring right away. When the body synchronizes with gravity, the task may seem to be completed without effort.

We feel heavy and uncomfortable as time appears to crawl while we are standing with our whole weight on one leg with a locked and misaligned knee joint. Similar to this, practice standing on both feet evenly while waiting in line at the bank, theater, or airport. Let your knees be soft and your body weight falls into your pelvis, legs, and feet. You may experience a rapid increase in your level of focus, awareness, and openness. Once you start to notice the little funny and colorful nuances that are present in practically every scene, your irritation and unhappiness will fade. Observe everything around you, take it all in, and be mindful of your surroundings while maintaining self-awareness. It seems as if you see the outside while looking inside. While you sit inside of yourself as if at home, this heightens your sensitivity.

It's feasible that sexual energy, or life energy, will increase in direct proportion as we put our internal vital energy circulation into practice. Take pleasure in feeling your body feel so alive. Sex is life's juice, therefore don't be frightened to experience it. You don't need to act on this energy to let it out. When you wait for love to enter your life, contain it, focus it inside you, and wait. Instead of seeking it out or anticipating it, welcome it. The simplest things may contain the greatest amounts of love, so look again.

Since our sexual energy is always looking for a way to express itself, the desire or drive for self-pleasure or masturbation may develop. Also, the need could signify a certain amount of internalized sexual tension or excitement. Yet it's vital to realize that masturbation is fertile ground for imagination, has nothing to do with reality, and maybe a distraction from awareness. Relaxation is a key component of making love, and self-pleasuring should be centered on this.

Guide yourself with the Love Keys. Keep any sexual tension or eagerness at bay while you touch and groom yourself. Stroke your legs, feet, and buttocks slowly and deliberately instead. Each lingering contact should be slowly reabsorbed. Your presence and experience will be more intense if you touch while also being aware of the contact. Roll around and enjoy your sensuality while taking long, deep breaths and spreading your energy throughout your body.

Continually touching oneself should be done if an orgasmic urge develops. The end is not something you should rush to. Be mindful of what is occurring as it occurs and let yourself get lost in the feeling when you ejaculate or have an orgasm. Put one hand on your heart if you can. It's best to refrain from invoking sexual imagery, but if it's required, a guy should try to picture his vagina or a woman her penis. This maintains the focus on the physical location of love—between the penis and vagina—rather than on vivid sexual fantasy, which is thrilling and provocative.

The desire for masturbation reportedly decreased, much to the astonishment of the men, following a period of conscious in-person sexual activity. The penis lost all inherent worth once sexual energy and the penis were seen as energy producers.

Begin a new relationship in consciousness

Explain that you want to try something new if you meet someone and want to make out. Even though it may seem a little intimidating, moving forward with it is best. Your sexual life will have a much better chance of developing into love if you can start it with a conscious component. In addition, women must start making intentional decisions and cease making concessions to males since they pay a price for doing so.

However, the mind will make an effort to keep you from talking about it for a while and persuade you to do it the traditional way. The emotional reactions brought on by unconscious sex, however, are frequently so quick, unpredictable, and overwhelming that we frequently part ways before we even realize it! Because sexual energy is misunderstood and has repercussions, love is not given the chance to blossom, let alone get off the ground.

As everyone has a vulnerability within, don't be hesitant to bring up the issue of sex. That is perplexing to us all. Talking about our emotions and having sex in public is often a relief and a way to relax. Provide an overview of what you've learned so far and offer ideas for a fresh approach. Find out which of the Love Keys you may utilize right away as you discuss them. To prevent excitement or focusing on a climax, begin slowly and take your time. I've been astonished by people's reactions to relaxing.

My acquaintance, who formerly reveled in switching lovers, once described to a new lady how he wanted to make love to her: very slowly, with eye contact, and without excitement or climax. Amazing outcomes were achieved! Every time, a huge gap opened in her body and heart, and she fell head over heels in love with him. A woman is particularly sensitive to the immense force of the love produced by a sentient penis, which is immediate and has unmatched intensity. She only sometimes has this awareness experience, so when she does, she is aware of it and wants more of it. The first penetration may be all that is necessary for her to feel satisfied and encountered. Similarly to this, a guy can never completely be satisfied by anything else once he experiences his sexual energy as a heavenly moving force.

It is common for partners in a relationship to feel the need to "have some space" or go out on their own for a bit because they see their partner's behavior as demanding, needy, or draining. Couples remark that this imbalance alters and there comes a satisfaction with silent and calm periods between them, with each one more centered and at home, as if they were alone together. This occurs when the attention of the lovemaking is directed inside and away from habitual orgasms.

- Vital energy can be circulated in the body while alone.
- Resting in consciousness is profoundly relaxing and rewarding.
- Energize the positive poles with the awareness.
- Most Love Keys can be used in daily life to great effect.
- When you meet someone new, start experimenting right away.

CHAPTER TWENTY SIX

THE LOVE TEMPLE

You may be reminded of the sanctity of romantic love by a room's ambiance, aroma, and taste. It could have an aura about it that inspires veneration and affection. It could serve as a reminder that you are here out of love, for love, and to love. You will quickly start to feel a wave of amazement and sensuality sweep through you when entering a bedroom that has been designed with lovemaking in mind with the bed as the main point. If you're going on a date where you want to make out, cleanse and tidy the space a few hours beforehand while giving it a loving touch. The environment will then be like a shrine, ideal for a celebration of love.

If you have the luxury of an extra room, make it your temple of love and save it for these special occasions. Remove as much of the furniture as you can, along with old mementos like portraits and photos. The goal is to provide a serene expanse that will help and encourage you into the clarity of the present moment. Take anything out of your bedroom that you don't need if you don't have any additional space. Generate the impression of a vacant area. Space might seem crowded, stuffy, or disorganized when ornaments and family photos accumulate dust and eventually fade into the background.

Your area will seem larger and give you a sensation of expansion if there are fewer items in it. My class was attended by an Italian couple who had been together for 25 years. As they got back home, they realized they needed to rearrange their furnishings to create a more supportive atmosphere for their renewed dedication to love. They were able to see one other once more by clearing away the unnecessary clutter of family relics.

Create a special atmosphere to make love

It's nice to have a variety of alternatives since lighting can make a huge impact in a space. Use four or five different lights of various hues to create a soft, cozy impression while making sure you have enough light to see your partner's eyes. It is initially simpler to be present when you can see one other, even if it might be lovely to make love in the closeness of darkness occasionally. Even when other lights are on at the same time, candlelight always has a unique effect on the environment. Use plenty of candles if you decide to stick to that, which is also extremely lovely so that the space is completely covered with dancing flames.

Before and during a romantic encounter, soft music helps to relax you and warms your heart. Put on a song you both like and let it loop until the passionate exchange is complete. Here is where auto-reverse CD and cassette players come in useful.

But, there are advantages to having a silent relationship. Music, I've discovered, may also serve as a screen and a place to lose oneself. Making love in silence is also beneficial since the consciousness is physically driven into the body, even though at first, it may seem strange without noises to encourage and support you.

The larger the better, a giant bed or a huge mattress on the floor is ideal so you can roll about and be fun without feeling awkward. Split-level postures, where one is sprawled out the half on and half off the bed, are ideal on low, big mattresses, giving one a somewhat feline sense. You may move around in rotational positions together on a bed with plenty of room, which improves genital communion and penetration depth. It's a good idea to choose a firm mattress so that your bodies have a stable base. It will be tough to discover and hold various postures if the mattress is excessively soft and collapses in the center.

Let your bed be an ongoing invitation that you can't reject since you both need to be properly supported and comfy. Slipping into a bed can be an exquisite and sensual experience when you have beautiful bed sheets, in terms of design, color, and quality. Moreover, keep a lot of pillows on hand so you may use them to support various body parts when you are having a romantic relationship. To increase the level of her pelvis and enable deeper penetration, a woman might, for instance, position a cushion under her hips while lying on her back. A cushion beneath the woman's buttocks may make the genital contact more intense and pleasant if you're having sex while sitting up, with her legs wrapped over your partner's hips (the Yab Yum position). Similar to how heads, necks, and legs sometimes need additional support.

The atmosphere is made more aesthetically pleasing and colorful by plants and flowers. Fill the space with a profusion of vibrant flowers, particularly roses that speak to the heart, if you and your partner are planning a special night, such as an anniversary or other occasion. Although maybe serve as a reminder to breathe more freely and deeply, the scent aids in maintaining your feeling of awareness. Incense, fragrant lamps, and candles may provide a distinct dimension to space since fragrance can be sensed when the space envelops the body. When there is incense burning, I always feel as if I am being enveloped by the environment. After a few instances, a certain aroma will start to be connected to love, and when you enter the room, you'll sense an openness within, a great ready-for love.

To reflect and intensify the surroundings, mirrors have long been a favorite feature in a space. It is quite OK to appreciate the reflection of your relaxed body and those of your partner in a mirror; it is even lovely. Yet, you should be aware that mirrors might pique your sexual inclinations. Using mirrors to let in more outside light is preferable. A view may be obtained twice or even more by positioning a mirror in front of a window. The positioning of mirrors allowed me to create the appearance of 88 flames from only 11 candles once. Use strips of mirror, anywhere from two to six inches broad, with a pencil-thick space between them as opposed to a single entire mirror, which is cumbersome and difficult to manage.

This has the wonderful effect of breaking up the reflection, enhancing it, and bringing up a whole new visual realm within your bedroom. Do whatever appeals to you, whatever seems magical and sensual, so that when you enter your room, the flickering candles and soothing music will remind you of a temple: tranquil, silent, fragrant, and flower-filled.

To make love in awareness, which needs a descent into the senses, prepare the body as you prepare your surroundings. Forget about the day's events and worries. The nicest thing one can do before making love is taking a warm shower or a soothing hot bath, and if they are feeling very daring, end with a sprinkle of cool water. Water is amazing because it cleanses your energy and makes you feel more present in both your body and soul. It also removes stale, clogged energy. To bring attention to the body, some movement, breathing exercises, and calm meditation are all beneficial.

With a namaste, you may begin and wonderfully end your love-making. The palms are joined in a posture of prayer and are held in front of the heart to make the traditional Indian hand gesture. A modest head-bobbing occurs in tandem with it.

This motion, often referred to as the heart mudra and activating the heart center, has the traditional meaning of "I welcome the Buddha in you." Sit across from one another, eyes in contact, and bow before starting to make love. Bow your heads in gratitude for the gifts that arise from being present while acknowledging each other and yourself. By doing so, you become more conscious of your surroundings.

You will often find yourself doing this heart mudra on the spur of the moment after an intensely passionate sexual encounter as a way of expressing your thanks to your partner. The reaction is practically automatic. When true love has been created, joy and tranquility beyond all comprehension come. When you gracefully tie the knot, enjoy the calm that follows.

Some individuals like rituals since they may assist them to create an original and unique environment for romantic engagement. Ritual acts as a portal that opens up to a set of instructions that invite you to engage your body and your senses in experiencing the present moment. It doesn't work for everyone, but for some, rituals or practices may be highly effective in creating an energy field to support their presence, so you might want to come up with your unique method of being ready for love. When you repeatedly follow this pattern, the rituals or practice's effects will start to reverberate in your body and get you ready for an inner trip.

Let grace fill your surroundings wherever you are with your priceless presence. Let your body be a perpetual reminder of the awareness that may be added to sex and love. A person may discover God inside themselves via sex, which is the greatest gift in life. The body is the most beautiful temple on earth.

KEY POINTS:

- Beauty and fragrant surroundings invoke the senses and inspire you.
- Design yourself a dream bed so it is a constant invitation to love.
- Use lighting, music, flowers, and fragrance to create ambience.
- The body is the greatest temple when radiant with presence.

The following meditation can be used as a preparation for lovemaking or to bring lovers closer when there is a feeling of separation.

CIRCLE OF LIGHT BREATHING — MEDITATION ON LIGHT

One of the oldest Tantra practices is a meditation on light. Something inside of you that has been a bud begins to open its petals as soon as you focus on the light during meditation. The opening of it is made possible by light meditation.

With flowers, music, and incense, turn your space into a shrine.

Lighting the space with candles will allow you to see your lover's eyes.

Place a mattress on the floor in the middle of the space with pillows at either end so that people may sit across from one another.

Place one candle in the space between the two cushions.

To sit comfortably and have the candle between you, make sure there is adequate room between the cushions.

Around 45 minutes of music should be chosen that opens and extends your energy.

Put extra cushions or seats far from the center of the room, toward the opposite ends.

The room should be prepared in advance and left unoccupied for 30 minutes while music is played.

After a shower, meet your partner in quiet at the temple's entrance wearing loose, comfortable attire that you may later take off if you choose.

Start the cassette or CD you've selected to listen to, or just leave it playing when you go in.

Slowly make your way to the two seats or cushions at the room's opposite ends, where you may sit in meditation for 10 to fifteen minutes.

Let a sense of serenity develop inside as you close your eyes. Put yourself in the spotlight and ignore your partner.

Bring your awareness into your belly and down your spine. Inhale till your navel is two inches below your nose.

Count to three as you exhale. Count to three as you inhale. Keep focusing on your stomach.

Breathe in this manner for many minutes.

Let your eyes open as soon as you sense yourself "arriving" in your body.

Let a delicate, introspective gaze, as if the temple were gazing directly into you. Feel your legs and feet like roots to the earth as you slowly get up.

To awaken the energy inside, bring a deep focus to the penis (for men) and breasts (for women).

Go cautiously in the direction of the place of worship.

Walking more slowly will help you experience your body more as energy than as a body.

On the mattress, take a seat across from one another and gaze at the candle flame.

Imagine that you are breathing in light when you inhale.

The lady is exhaling via her heart while inhaling through her vagina. The male breaths in via the heart and exhales through the penis.

Let the light go synchronistically through your body as you breathe out as if your lover is communicating with you.

Raise your eyes to meet your lover's and exchange energy via the eyes when you feel yourself being filled with light.

The lady travels across the room to sit in the Yab Yum posture after the guy has removed the candle from between you.

Breathe in synchronization as you continue to circulate the light, the lady in through your vagina and out through your heart, and the male in through your heart and out through your penis.

Breathe normally and keep the light moving until the music stops. When the time is right, softly part ways and adore your partner while saying "namaste" to express your appreciation (bow).

Make love or just relax by lying together.

CONCLUSION

Sex is one of the acts provided by God and nature in which you are continually thrust into the present. Even when you are making love, which is just for a little period, you are never in the present in everyday life. To decipher sex, according to the Tantra, one must comprehend it. There must be more to sexual activity if life is created as a result of it. The path to Divinity and God lies in that something greater.

I made a self-promise to keep when I first felt the need to write a book that it would be brief. The fundamentals of sex, while very complicated in implications, are elementary, which is how I felt at first and have felt more and more since. The majority of what I had seen about sex didn't seem at all uncomplicated. It seemed like I would have to put more effort into finding more. I came to see that doing less led to finding more. Sex is very easy since the male and female human bodies are exquisitely and cleverly designed to join, one flowing into the other with the ability to produce a heavenly biological ecstasy, raising us very effortlessly into the realm of love and meditation, a need for spiritual renewal.

Similar to how we depend on oxygen and water, we need sex. We feel like an empty shell, dragging the rigid body, tired in the soul, and sad in the heart without this vital vitality flowing within. Sex is our connection to the divine, the secret to energy alchemy, and the key to unlocking the secrets of life.

Being able to create this euphoric energy in awareness is a benefit of being a human, and it is this consciousness that sets humans apart from other animals. Animals do not have an "awareness" of themselves; they are ecstatically present to the glory of the moment only in instinct, even though humans may learn a lot by seeing them engage in love play. This may have persuaded us to reject sex as a spiritless, just instinctual animal behavior. We fulfill our animal nature via reproduction, which is the falling part of the sexual energy cycle. Nevertheless, we also embody the rising spiritual phase, which is characterized by the formation of ecstatic sexual energy.

As a consequence of ubiquitous indoctrination that has devalued sex, we have been denied access to its ecstatic spiritual side. As sex is superficially seen as a physical or emotional requirement, we are hesitant to bring it up in conversation when our emotions are mixed, so we seem to be disinterested in it. Other obsessions and compulsions take root as a result of our disregard for sex. We are nonetheless motivated, nevertheless, by sex's subliminal forces. It's necessary for us to "do it" sometimes, and when it is, we keep it a secret.

Traffic is decreased and a short-term objective is accomplished, but real love is not experienced sexually. I've heard from some guys who claim that when they were initially getting into a relationship, their instinct was to lay within the genital area. They wanted to do it. After that, they were shocked and forced themselves to turn painfully away from their pleasant nature by watching movies, listening to rumors, reading publications, and engaging in forced effort in sex.

According to what I've seen, people connect with their innocence more readily when they are younger since they are better able to ignore or reject the effects of our sexual indoctrination. Nevertheless, as the years go by, the protective layer of conditioning that is thrown about us becomes harder, our anxieties intensify, our tensions take on a physical shape, resignation sets in, we become used to our routines, and complacency keeps us bound to many unconscious habits. The fact that awareness is all that is necessary for this sexual mistake to be resolved is what makes it so beautiful.

The earlier we can begin, the better. Only a select few strong people have the good fortune to be what may be described as "naturally Tantric" and to preserve this divinely endowed sexual purity throughout their whole lives, while others only need one great Tantric experience to profoundly alter their life. Others may experience a steady erosion, a gentle transition from darkness to light, and an enjoyable journey through all the forms and textures in between as they attempt to reclaim this sexual simplicity.

I could only dispel misconceptions about making love via physical contact. The difference was created by really doing it rather than just thinking about it or discussing it. It is quite different to talk about how you want to make love than to do it while keeping that promise. When the bodies have come together, these unconscious habits start to come into play, and we might discover that the values we initially had may not be so simple to uphold. In the beginning, our presence and awareness are not nearly as powerful as the unconscious forces in the body, and they are tenacious. We are in the place we are. It involves learning to connect outside of the immediate sexual experience and bringing the sexual experience gradually into awareness. Soon after, if not before I was penetrated, the impulse to "go for coming" would strike me.

It took me some time to change my thoughts and disconnect from the physical reflexes that were pulling me down the track automatically since my body and brain were so used to reacting to the impulse. My body gradually learned how to react naturally to each moment as my interest in orgasm faded, allowing me to discover that every experience was different.

It is necessary to repeatedly make love to the same person to put these changes in awareness into action and transform your love experience on a qualitative level. Two wonderful instruments are gradually tuned to one another, resulting in beautiful harmony. The magnetic poles align and ecstatically melt into one another as finesse develops over time.

Couples must be committed to it since it seldom occurs by chance unless you are fortunate. It's as if there's a switch that has to be switched on, which is the easiest thing in the world, but we've lost the knack, so we need practice. The commitment must, above all, be made to the present, to this moment, and not to the next. I had no option but to make love at this very moment since when I initially started exploring, it was a daily thing. I might claim that this improved my awareness since it compelled me to remain in the present, made me feel urgent, and prevented me from wasting a chance. Not tomorrow, but right now, I had to make love as sensually and purposefully as I could. It never gets better.

To start over again, you must have the following qualities: adaptability, amusement, willingness to change, and a willingness to be flexible. Embrace a fresh new approach to exploring who you are. Having the confidence to try, to exchange experiences while making love, and to discuss it afterward is necessary if you want to allow this to develop inside and educate yourself as a couple. Maybe even with specificity. Every degree of closeness you attain with your partner will be mirrored in your lovemaking, which will become more sensitive and enjoyable.

Do not forget to pay attention to your physical and emotional reactions to making love, as well as how connected you feel to your partner. You will start to get answers to these inner inquiries that will help you understand the fundamental purpose of romantic love and how to keep harmony and love in your life. It can seem like you are getting your first sight of what love is all about. Experience is where real learning occurs. While you're "blissed out," you can be sour and miserable the following.

Why? Why were you so unhappy with lovemaking, exactly? What actions did you take, and how were they taken? You may gradually start to increase the sex's level of awareness by using this as a guide. An effective method to dispel the shadows is to be aware of the effects of our sexual encounters. When we can see how our unconscious selves manifest in sex, it motivates us to change it right away via awareness. With our intellect, we gradually shed light on something that had previously been buried in mystery.

We experience this change via transition, developing into a distinctive sexual expression by navigating our path and laying the experienced groundwork. No amount of lofty ideas, impatience, anxiety, or switching from one strategy to another will help. With the rigidity of constraint meant to disguise ignorance, there is a risk of losing the innocent delight and sensuality of learning via physical experience.

The seeds of development may be found in actual uncertainty and shakiness. You will be supported into a more straightforward, nourishing, and loving experience of love if you use the Love Keys as a guide. These are useful tips to help you infuse your body with awareness and a sense of immediate connection, which shows sex as a new and enlivening experience.

Couples often perceive their attitude toward sexual exploration incorrectly, according to what I have seen. In doing so, the traditional and Tantric approaches to sex are being distinguished. The one is focused on movement and climax, while the second embraces slowness and quiet, and this is the first superficial distinction between the two. Couples will therefore determine that this is the main focus of their relationship. Before initiating a sexual act, they will determine how they want to proceed. Even though the value of a few minutes of stillness and silence is not to be lightly dismissed, in the long run, this method creates a division and a subsequent lack of integration within the body and psychology of each person. "Today, are we going to be still and silent according to Tantra, or shall we do it in the old way with movement and excitement?" By having both a soft half and a hard portion, it strengthens our dualism.

The development of the poles' magnetic characteristics is greatly impeded and the poles experience confusion on an energy level as well. The genital organs are required to be both demanding and robust, as well as sensitive and responsive on one hand. Since one stride forward means two steps back, this duality itself creates tension, preventing the fundamental roots of awareness from taking hold. Which way to make love—this manner or that way? is posed in this statement. rather than enabling the body's intellect to develop via conscious trial and error.

Tantra demands the whole of you, not just either/or choices. It wants all of your motion, ecstasy, orgasms, calm, inner concentration, and awareness together. Your sexual energy will be permanently changed by a comprehensive re-education in sex. Both on a personal and interpersonal level, this occurs. It is still considered personal progress when one's sensitivity grows as a result of developing awareness. The joint process has already been very beneficial to each individual, even if a couple decides to split.

Even when a partnership or romantic connection ends, the awareness ingrained in the penis and vagina persists. External factors do not affect awareness since consciousness is consciousness. You will be quickly noticed by your next lover. Once awareness is realized, there is no other way to experience love since it is so much more full and incorporates everything.

A beautiful reality of movement emerges during meditation. Integration occurs at a fundamental level via the merging of sex and spirit. But this is not a transition that happens as a result of separation, choosing a certain direction for love today, or even, as I was once informed, making love one way in the mornings and another way in the afternoons! The sexual integrity of the body is overridden if one chooses in advance with the mind which direction to make love with the body, and the genitalia need time to build their magnetic finesse.

Tantra is a call to mindfulness and awareness in every act of making love. To be as present and attentive as possible, let that be the beginning point at all times. Everything of it. This is a good beginning. It doesn't matter where it goes or how it turns out; what matters is where you are right now—where your awareness is. Tantra emphasizes how you behave rather than what you do. The goal of the bow is to bring consciousness to sex by experiencing every moment as it passes minute by minute and by being present with whatever is going on within the body.

We must confront our previous routines, desires, and cravings since the body houses our history and extensive individual and societal programming. At the same time as we consciously meet and welcome our wants, we also keep a closer eye on what is going on. It is comparable to viewing a movie in which you are the main character while seeing it from behind a camera. You continue to be aware of the actions being taken, the shallower breathing, and the way the sexual energy is consciously increased until the peak sensation and then released.

You will naturally slow down as a result of this mindfulness, which will also help you stay on the road and increase your enjoyment via its generosity. Just start paying attention to what you're doing while having fun. Sexual energy can't gradually change and react in a way that is deeply anchored in the body; that is only possible when you are conscious of everything you do.

Repressing your conditioning has the potential of causing you to lose your authenticity, which will have an impact on both you as a pair and as an individual. This is another disadvantage of the replacement strategy. Avoiding all excitement may work for a time if you can change that "how" via knowledge and mindfulness, but sooner or later you will probably find yourself yawning and feeling the desire to go to sleep. The sex energy will not be one of expanding into it and giving in to its higher intellect, of being extended and alive in it; even if the connection between the penis and vagina may feel pleasant, the experience will be one lacking in challenge.

During making love, you could start to miss the thrill and feel restless. This restlessness may be expressed as a want for activity, a need to move or to come, or a desire to abandon everything and return to the old ways. One should anticipate this. As a result of your denial, your unconsciousness is banging on your back door. Your sexual energy is now where you believe it should be because you rejected where you are and put a notion on it. It is not a repressive denial that the unconscious requires, but a conscious expression. For it to gradually become aware, you must dance with it and travel with it.

To explore the mystery of sex, a couple must dance consciously between the old and the new, and coming face to face with their unconscious selves becomes an adventure. To capture the moment when one has lost awareness or gone forward out of the realm of the present, the technique involves coming back to the present moment again and over again. The core cord is a thread of consciousness that, like a shuttle, moves back and forth between being aware of awareness lapses and being aware of awareness itself, strengthening consciousness and bringing the present to the fore.

Be mindful of your surroundings at all times. Once we let go of the built-up tensions in sex and liberate it from a constrained course, it develops into a flexible, creative dynamic force. The secret is to cultivate awareness, keep observing, and over time you will see that harmony and balance are gently developing within you.

For the energy to flow upward, which is the normal direction for it to move, we must draw it within. Streaming phenomena will start to be felt in the center of the body, beginning from the genitals and running upward into the heart and head.

Pleasure now takes on a new dimension and transforms into a euphoric full-body experience thanks to this inversion of sexual energy. A luminous, tingling, orgasmic cellular vibration may first be extremely mild or only felt in certain locations. A golden highway is forming its way up the body as this streaming sensation becomes stronger.

Practice makes inward turning easier, and the electromagnetic joy produced by the polarity of the penis and vagina rises upward. It is possible to force oneself into the present with the Love Keys. This demonstrates that you are approaching your goal of bringing awareness to your body with a powerful attitude and clear purpose. The change in consciousness is really strong. These basic energies flow more freely when there is an intensity of present, availability to the moment, and openness to oneself and your partner. As the sexual core is relaxed, it goes upward while gaining a lot of energy.

This is the recycling or recirculation of the sexual energy, which recirculates back to the brain, where it originated, flashing through the body's center. The body becomes an instrument with a melodic inner flute that can react to finer and finer rhythms spiraling upward, the energy taking an exhilarating trip to access the higher centers. The perception of sex as a heavenly experience continues to expand as the polarity strengthens, causing the organs of love to produce euphoric sexual energy.

It is an awareness of a silent, calm, intensely captivating interior phenomenon. Silence breaches the barrier, and a miracle melting takes place—the outside man combines with his inner woman, and the outer woman merges with her inner man—as a man and a woman grow and rise in love. This resonance strengthens the internal rod of magnetism in each body's opposite pole. This orgasmic union of a man and a female is euphoric love, awakening the mechanism of our inner celebration.